THE HUNGER DIARIES

OR: HOW TO LOSE WEIGHT FASTING AND EATING WELL

The Hunger Diaries, or:
How to Lose Weight Fasting and Eating Well

Written by Andrew Mackay

Edited by Aly Quinn

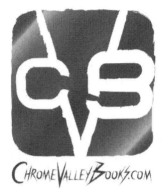

CHROMEVALLEYBOOKS.COM

ISBN: 9781081305864
Copyright © 2019 Chrome Valley Books

IMPORTANT NOTICE:

~ Acknowledgments ~

My wonderful advance reader team.
Jennifer Long and Adele Embrey.
Dr. Jason Fung, Jimmy Moore,
and Thomas DeLauer.
Everyone who wants to incinerate their body fat
within a reasonable delay.
I love you all.

MENU

Introduction

"… unless you can find an eating program you can stay on for the rest of your life, dieting is a waste of time."
- Roger Ebert, May 7th, 2004.

I'm going to make a prediction.

You are overweight or obese.

Am I right? I don't know for sure because I can't see you.

If you're *not* overweight or obese then the odds are that you're reading this book for fun, or you're interested in the subject. That's fine, too. This book has something for everyone (probably, I guess we'll see when I've written it?).

In any event, let's get back to *you* (yes, you!) - the person who's either "looking inside" at Amazon to preview the book to see if you should buy it (answer: yes, you should) or, better yet, the kind soul who's paid less than the price of a full-fat latte and bagel meal deal at *Bean There, Done That* - the fictitious version of *Starbucks* you'll be hearing more about in the coming pages - in order to have acquired this masterpiece.

Either way, you're interested in how to shred a few (or a truckload of) pounds.

I have some terrific news for you. I promise you're going to love it. Over the past forty years of my life I've developed a psychological technique that smashes barriers to progress. Anyone can adopt it because, quite honestly, you're probably already very good at it anyway and you just don't realize it. Yet.

The phrase you're about to digest (hoho!) is vital for your journey. It's something I've developed, and it's called *(drum roll…)*

FOOL YOURSELF

Here's the thing.

If, like me, you are overweight or obese, then you've already mastered the art of ***Fool Yourself***. I'm sure some of you are already way ahead of me, but allow me to explain.

You've spent the past few weeks / months / years waddling around *believing* everyone thinks you're not overweight because you:

1: Wear baggy clothes.

2: Sport a beard to hide your droopy chin / neck.

3: Avoid mirrors and reflective surfaces to prevent reminders of "just how disgusting you are." Seriously, you are *really* good at this one, and don't deny it.

4: Look in the mirror out of unavoidable necessity (i.e. application of make-up, shaving, brushing your teeth). You may not realize it, but you tilt your head / body to finally settle on an acceptable angle of yourself and decide you're not *that bad looking*, after all.

How do I know this? Because, frankly, I do the same. Actually, scratch that. EVERYBODY DOES IT.

Isn't it a relief to know you're not alone?

Just accepting where you are - that's one hurdle smashed before we've started. Only a few more to go...

However, before you get all depressed, allow me to introduce you to *the good part*. Because you're such an expert at **Fool Yourself**, you possess *precisely* the mental skill and ability to make this fat-shredding exercise a resounding success.

Oh, believe me, we're going to go into laser-sharp precision on why **Fool Yourself** is important. I won't spoil it here, but it's going to naturally ferment throughout the diary. If you're old (like me) you may remember the days as a kid when Diet "Soda" didn't exist. You only drank full-fat, regular "Soda", and then "Diet Soda" came out, and most of us fatties began to drink it. We believed for a few weeks that we were drinking the real thing because - hey - it's *Diet*, right? Some magical potion invented by the <name removed on legal advice> company that incinerates fat just by consuming it. Before long, we fooled ourselves that it was good for us (or at least better than the original) so much we began to believe it. Today, we've made "Diet Soda" the best-selling soda on the planet - bar none.

That's just a sneak peek into the whole ***Fool Yourself*** mindset, which I'll expand on very soon.

*** * ***

If you are *not yet thin* (mindset is everything, my portly friend lol) then I'm going to make a list of reasons why that is. You want to lose weight. Yeah, you and everyone else. But wait. Let me guess *why* you want to lose weight:

1: You want to be more attractive to the opposite / same sex (e.g. get someone into bed).

2: You've been dieting intermittently all your life - only to pile the pounds back on, you mischievous *yo-yo*-er, you.

3: You've had a health scare, or maybe (Heaven forbid) something worse. Your doctor demands you change your ways or risk injury and / or death.

You'll notice the order of the above-mentioned list is important.

I'm generalizing, of course. Lots of you reading this work of genius will certainly be doing it for at least one of the above-mentioned reasons. But, for the majority of you, reason #1 is at the top of the list quite without chance. Now, I *could* tell you why "being more attractive" (despite your age) is at #1. However, I think it's far more powerful if *you* arrive at the answer yourself.

Before we do that, I want to reintroduce you the word "attractive". It doesn't mean you want to sleep with someone. It means, quite simply, pleasant to be around.

Okay, I want you to close your eyes (not yet, keep reading the instructions) and cook up an image of a *very* obese person. Man or woman, or even a child. Let's keep it easy for now and suggest it's someone you *don't* know. Make sure the image in your mind is big, like an IMAX screen.

Close your eyes **now**.

So, you've seen the image? All I'm going to ask you is one question:

Which ONE adjective springs to mind when you see that image?
Don't over think it.
I want the first word that popped into your mind.

Okay, so you have a word. My guess is you thought of one of the following:

Ugly, gross, disgusting, nasty, avoid, eurgh, yuck, no, death / die, or *fat*.

Was I right?

Meh. It doesn't matter if I was. According to the *Institute of Mackay Predictions*, statistically, 92.2% of you thought of one of those words or very similar, and that leaves you remaining 7.3% of the population thinking the opposite. Something along the lines of "Aww, bless their artery-clogged heart, I feel sorry for you," or, worse yet, "I see this every damn day, so it's no big deal."

Now imagine that very same person you conjured up in your mind's eye approaches *you* to:

1 - Ask you on a date.

2 - Interview for a position at your company.

3 - Sit next to you in economy class on a budget airline.

Be brutally honest. How do you feel about them, now? The chances are that if you're perfectly okay with *any* of those three, then… (drum roll)… you're obese, yourself.

You won't do this, and, frankly, I don't advise it. *But…* if you were to ask a person of optimal weight for their height then their answer to the above is likely to cause offense.

Fear not, dear reader. Help is at hand…

… which I'll get to in just a moment.

Now, see that Roger Ebert quote you read right at the top of the introduction?

I want you to remember it.

Actually, scratch that. Remembering it is good but it's not enough. I want you to type the quote into a word processor in a big-ass font and print it out and stick it to your wall. Preferably just above your oven, or just out of *eyeshot* at your work station, or wherever you spend most of your time.

Heck, print five copies.

Because unless you read, absorb, comprehend, process, and finally, just *apply* the quote as gospel (thanks, *Bloom's Taxonomy*!), then you may as well stop reading here. Go get a refund and ask for your money back, or pass this copy of the book to someone who *will* accept the quote and respect it.

Sorry to be so prescriptive and indelicate. It's in my nature. I like to think that what you're about to read is funny and somewhat yucky in places but, at the very least, *informative*. Food for thought, if you will.

There aren't too many books out there that chronicle a ~~diet~~ journey of this nature. Day by day. With such brutal honesty. I'm about to bare my soul here, warts and all. There are some books like this, but not to put too fine a point on it, *they're not written by anyone as imaginative and stupid as I am.*

Which leads me nicely onto…

Just Who ~~Does~~ is Andrew Mackay ~~Think he is,~~ Anyway?

Funny you should ask that.

Who do I think I am?

I think I'm a bit like you; fat, and with a fast-food-to-healthy-eating ratio which will probably send my actuary tables crashing down.

Just to be sure, let's back this up with evidence. At time of writing (Saturday, June 22nd) here's the lowdown:

<u>My height:</u>
5'11" / 61.32 inches

<u>*My weight:*</u>
15.5 stone / 217 lbs / 98.4 kg

<u>My waist size:</u>
40" (UK)

<u>My Body Mass Index (BMI):</u>
29.99
(Patient.info)

30.2
(NHS UK)

It's a well-known fact that a BMI of 30+ means you're *obese*. The healthy, acceptable range is in the lower twenties, depending on your height.

Riiiight. This is interesting. According to the Americans, I'm teetering on the edge of obesity at a frightening 29.9 BMI. According to my geographical brethren at the National Health Service (NHS) I *am* obese; clocking in at an unfortunate *0.2* past the 30 BMI threshold of obesity.

What this tells me is that I definitely need a range of reputable sources reporting back to me when I'm fact-checking anything.

Damn, man. I'm technically obese. How the hell did that happen?

How Andrew Mackay Got Obese.

I was a chubby kid growing up – thanks in part to my mother's home cooking - but also because school lunch was mostly soda, fries and cake. My mother isn't to blame. Every mother cooked at home. McDonald's was a treat. I am a child of the eighties, way before bulk buying and nutritional labels on every food was a thing. I don't recall much (about anything, honestly) in the way of options for school meals. Certainly no fruit or vegetables. It was all-but impossible to avoid the ice cream van / candy store on the way home. I was never very sporty, either. And so it was that little Andrew Mackay wasn't so little - at least horizontally. Never *obese*, but hardly the desire of others.

In 2006, I experienced my first bout of severe back pain. Since then I've "thrown my back out" about seven times doing the simplest of things; reaching up to grab something off the shelf being the first culprit. Even sneezing, washing my hands in the basin, and turning awkwardly in bed the stupidest little movement, and it's all over. Each time I'm in severe pain and of no use to man nor beast for about a week. Of course, this is weight-related.

Now that I've put the violin away, let's see where I am on the official "*Chub-o-Meter.*" I want to know where *I should be at*, according to two valid sources of health information, one British, the other American. For my height…

Target Weight Range:
9 stone, 6 lbs - 12 stone 11 lbs
(134.4 lbs - 168.54 lbs)
(61 kg - 76.9 kg)

Okay. I need to lose 50 lbs to reach my optimum / recommended weight. I need hit 12 stone *on the nose*, or 167 lbs, or 76 kg. If we're rounding up the over / under, then this is the target I should be striving for.

Yippee! I now have my ONLY goal which I'll refer to as "Goal #1" or "My Only Goal." One goal at a time. I can't shed 50 lbs in two weeks. That's just silly. I'll figure out a reasonable deadline to reach for later, but first…

- Some Interesting Facts AboutYour New, Favorite Author -
Andrew Mackay Esq, Ba (Hons), PGCE

Before I became a self-published Amazon best-selling author, I used to be a teacher. The stress alone would kill me. I hardly slept or had any time for myself. The kids' behavior got worse by the year. I rarely ate at work, and when I did, it was intermittent and mostly unhealthy. I was angry, confused, upset, and well into depression. Who knows what might have happened if I continued?

Since gouging the metaphorical malignant tumor that is teaching out of my life back in the summer of 2016, I put on weight due to the sedentary lifestyle of a typical author. I use my car a lot more, for one thing. After a number of best-sellers, the money was mostly spent on takeout food of some description. I love food and so does my wife. To protect her anonymity, I'll refer to her as "Amelia."

Our relationship is *somewhat* based on food - or at least it feels that way, sometimes.

She and I love it all - McDonald's, KFC, Doner Kebabs (US version: Giros), French Fries, Indian, Chinese, Japanese, Thai… I mean, the list goes on. Not that I kept a tally, but if I'm being brutally honest, I'd *guesstimate* that two out of every ten dinners we have eaten in our mid-to-late twenties and thirties has been takeout. Lots of "Diet Soda" (or variants) too.

It's a small miracle that I haven't developed an illness, gangrene, or gone blind by now at the tender age of forty. On that last point about blindness, I do wear spectacles, but it's more for eyesight preservation because (shock, horror!) as an author, I'm at my computer screen more often than I'm not.

I also smoke approximately one pack of cigarettes a day, which - I gather - will actually help matters. They're an appetite-suppressor. For Heaven's sake, do not *start* smoking. I'm not proud of some of the things I've done in my life but taking up smoking was the worst decision ever. In any event, now isn't the time to quit. Not yet, anyway.

There is a small history of Type 2 diabetes in my family. I refuse to let this happen to me. Obesity aside I'm in reasonably good health. I'm not on any medication of any kind. I think I have a shot at shedding the pounds. Unfortunately, I also have breasts (I'll use the spoonerism "Titch Bits" for this) which is great if you're a cross-dresser or juggling drag queen act, but not if you're trying to achieve the unachievable levels of Adonis-properties I desire this week.

It's nice to meet you, too, by the way.

Who This Book is For.

It's really hard to tell right now. You see, I devised this plan today (Saturday, June 22nd) to lose weight. I just started typing an hour ago. I haven't quite thought this through, if I'm honest. What I *do* know is that if I burn more calories than I take in then I'll lose weight. That's about as mathematical and scientific as these diaries will get.

Absolutely none of this was in my mind when I woke up this morning. *None of it.* The idea for this dangerous adventure popped into my head about three hours ago. It was an impulsive decision. My life is ruled by impulse decisions. I live in "Chrome Valley", UK, and the decision to move here from London was impulsive. Quitting teaching was, essentially, an impulsive act. I met Amelia outside the college building one night by accident, and our first ever date was impulsive. Most of our decisions are. Also, we're waiting for news of our impending house move. The decision to sell up and move was impulsive, too. My decisions always will be, and don't get me started on last-minute decisions when I'm writing fiction. They're some of the best storytelling decisions I've ever made.

Much like you, I suspect, I'm not good at planning ahead or being organized. But I am ruthlessly determined and on first-name terms with my will power.

And so, without further delay, this book is for:

1: Serious weight-loss wannabes who have tried absolutely everything else and failed.

2: Someone hungry (sorry) for a no-holds-barred and unflinching account of a near-insane author putting his body and mind through the mincer - *all without medical advice or supervision.* Honestly, this idea is so stupid and dangerous, of that I am well aware, thanks. But I want to start now and not in another two months' time before I can get an appointment with my GP on the already-stretched NHS and gorge fifty-eight more half-pounders with bacon and cheese in the interim.

3: Someone who understands humor and a joke when they see it, doesn't take everything they read too literally, and does not trigger easily. I'm sure the topics of fat shaming, eating disorders, and other controversial themes will rear their heads at some point. Despite the inevitable use of PG-rated curse words, there will be jokes that will challenge some readers. Please take it in the satirical spirit it's intended. For posterity's sake, I need to document *the real me*, and not some fictionalized "nice" version of Andrew Mackay *you* want to read.

4: Someone who, by now, has remembered the opening quote by Roger Ebert verbatim in their mind, and simply accepts that - without it - all of this is a waste of time.

Ugh. Someone's going to take exception to something in this book. I just know it. This is such a controversial subject. Nevertheless, it's in my nature to lampoon and mock. *This is fair warning.*

Did you check *all four* on the list above?

If not, you can stop reading or continue on for entertainment purposes.

If, on the other hand, you *did* score 4 / 4, then congratulations! I believe you're in safe company. We'll get to the plan in a moment. Before we do, you and I can have a little fun reading the next section and have a giggle at those delusional, stay-forever-fat individuals who have given up already, stopped reading, and asked for a refund. Those people fit nicely into an important section I've aptly named:

Who This Book is NOT For.

This part is easy.

Before we get to the easily-digestible list, if you are an authority on nutrition (a doctor, physician, nutritionist, clinician, etc) then this book isn't aimed at you, but you may find it interesting, purely from an "in-the-moment" account from an (obese) layman who has no clue what he's doing but keen to learn, evolve, and adapt accordingly. No doubt you'll laugh at some of the theories. That's cool with me. I hope you choke laughing your ass off.

As for the rest of you, if any of the below applies to you, then just give up. Waddle away. No damage done. Well, not to me, anyway. No doubt we'll see you again when your cake-diet fails and you come scurrying back in a few years' time with a significantly-aged and rundown metabolism.

This book isn't for you if you:

1: Do not respect food.

2: Do not respect yourself or others.

3: Are only committed to a couple weeks / months to get the weight off, only to return to your old, cheeseburger-based ways and *re-blob*.

According to many, many health reports from reputable sources, there is a chance you are not able to lose weight by traditional means. A genetically disadvantaged metabolic rate, for example. However, the chances of someone in that unfortunate position are vanishingly small; *almost* as unlikely as the same people finding this book and actually reading it.

However, if you have medical evidence to support such a claim, then please read on. I don't want to discriminate in any way and I am sure you will find something helpful within these pages.

Still here? Wow, good for you. You've scored well. Hey, listen to me. *You* need to take a long, hard think about *why* you want to lose weight. Remember that opening quote from Roger Ebert? Of course you do. With that in mind, if your ultimate goal is to lose weight so that you can:

1: Get in the sack with someone you find hot…

2: Stop your partner / friends taking the piss about your "titch bits" or love handles…

3: Go back to your bucket of fried chicken five times per day after you've shed the weight…

… then guess what? This book ain't for you, either. Go away.

You're losing weight for *you*, and you alone.

It might be that now isn't the time for you, but you do take this seriously. That's cool - as long as you're realistic about this process and set your expectations accordingly.

Good. We've separated the boys from the men, if you'll forgive the hideously outdated and politically incorrect phrase.

Now, take your seats. The show is about to begin. I hope you're sitting comfortably - well, as comfortably as you can in that increasingly small chair you've managed to wedge your planet-sized buttocks into…

THE HUNGER DIARIES

— THE PLAN —

1: The Detail.

I want to reduce my appetite and reset my taste buds. Also, I want to reduce my daily calorie intake to near-dangerous levels and take up a modest amount of exercise. You know, *eat less, move more.* Everybody does it.

I've decided I'll eat one potato, one banana, one apple, one yogurt, one tin of tuna, and drink as many apple squashes (US version: "cordials") and coffees with whole milk (US version: "creamer") as I want, per day. I'm giving up the Diet Soda, too. The half-full tin is bubbling away on my desk as I type this very sentence, and it's somewhat angry with me for doing all this. Giving up chocolate and anything remotely bad for me is a no-brainer, obviously. It's worth noting that my wife and I have a few unopened tubes of Pringles, uneaten (Chunky) Kit Kats, and around ten tins of Diet Soda in the fridge, all waiting to tempt me into submission.

I won't be eating unhealthy / fast food, naturally.

Because we're in the middle of a heatwave (and will be for some time) in the UK, I'll go to bed around 3 am each night, and rise at 11 am. My bedroom cooks from the morning sun so I'd rather sleep through it.

I'll log the calorie count each day, along with a brutal play-by-play of each day revealing my physical and mental state.

I'll do this for fourteen days. A calendar fortnight. It's Saturday June 22nd as I write this. I'm going to start on Monday, June 24th. A brand new week, and my wife will be at work for twelve hours each weekday, so that'll be interesting.

Some or all of this could change. New information or research could come to light, and I have allowed myself the ability to adapt my plan on the condition that it is backed up with sufficient evidence from at least *three* different, quality, and trusted sources. After all, it's how the *eat less, move more* theory came into practice.

I am going in raw, as they say in Greece. *Probably.*

On the fifteenth day, Monday July 8th, I will finish this diary with a bang. After two weeks of potatoes and tuna I am closing the book on what it's like to finally consume one of my favorite dishes; a large lamb kebab and fries, garnished with cabbage and lettuce, and drenched in garlic mayonnaise and chili sauce. Call it a reward. Actually, let's call it… *Kebab Monday.*

2: Inspiration - Where the Idea Came From.

Although I kind of knew this already, the initial germ of the idea I had a few hours ago came from some trivia I read about a movie called *The Machinist*, starring Christian Bale. He plays a ridiculously underweight character who starts to hallucinate on his night shifts. The film wasn't great, but it was the radical weight loss that intrigued me. According to the trivia, Mr. Bale dropped from 173 lbs to 110 lbs - and for a tall guy, that's dangerously stupid. Way below target weight, if nothing else. How did he do it? A daily diet of one apple, one tin of tuna, and the occasional black coffee and an even rarer whiskey. He'd go on to pile all the pounds back on and muscle up for *Batman Begins* which began shooting six months later.

Next up, about an hour ago I watched a YouTube video called "How Penn Jillette Lost Over 100 lbs and Still Eats Whatever He Wants." I'll include a link to this, and all the other references, as an addendum at the back of the book. He talks about "The Mono Diet" where, for fourteen days straight, he only ate a baked or boiled potato whenever hunger set in. It's unclear how many times per day he did this but I am estimating over a sixteen-hour "awake" period he must have started with at least three. As the days progressed and his stomach and appetite shrank, he got by on *maybe* two potatoes, or one. He mentions that his taste buds reset themselves and, having previously been obese and gorging on bad food (i.e. *me* right now), he had a new-found appreciation for good, healthy food (certainly *not* me!).

In short, I'm going to combine both of those sources of inspiration, no matter how ill-advised (hence the term *inspiration*). I'll just refer to it as the Bale / Jillette *thing*. What is this *thing*, anyway? An experiment? A journey? An adventure? A diet? I dunno, but it's certainly *not the last one*. More on that towards the end of this chapter.

3: Preparation

It's now Sunday, June 23rd. Amelia and I went to a well-known supermarket to get a few tins of tuna, a bag of potatoes, some "low-fat", "no-added-sugar" yogurt, and apple squash (Cordial) to add to my tall glass of filtered water.

Lunch today occurred at around 2 pm. I had one ham and cheese sandwich on brown bread and half a tube of Jalapeno-flavored Pringles. This is the lunch I always have, although the flavor of the potato chips changes from time to time. I estimate lunch was somewhere in the region of 1,000 calories.

8 pm. Dinner. I had a Chicken Tikka Masala and Pilau rice, processed food that was microwaved. I had eight poppadums and two teaspoonfuls of mango chutney. I also had two, small nan breads to go with it. Again, a typical dinner for me when it *isn't* takeout.

For dessert I had a Chunky Kit Kat.

Dinner must have set me back somewhere in the region of 3,000 - 3,500 calories.

I do smoke, but I rarely have alcohol.

I am going to bed at around 2 am, and intend to wake up at 11 am, ready to start my adventure.

I've now decided a reasonable time frame for my only goal of reaching 12 stone / 167 lbs / 67 kg. My 41st birthday in October. Just over three months from now. In order to kick-start this long process, I need…

4: The Rules

Non-negotiable and I *must* adhere to them at all times.

This book is, first and foremost, written and designed for consumption by one person, and one person alone - *me*. It's my hope that documenting the next two weeks aids my quest to complete this journey. But, this is just the beginning. The first two weeks - my acclimation to a reduced appetite and desire for bad food - will undoubtedly be the hardest stretch of it all. The book cannot document a whole three months, otherwise it'd have to be in volumes like *Harry Potter*, and I'm not doing that. Anyway, if I ever need to undertake a diet in future, then a two-week record will be more than sufficient. I'm holding *nothing* back. No holds barred. I want a reminder of what to expect, how I felt and, hopefully, learn why I gained all that weight back.

Thus, I undertake a list of non-negotiable "vows".

I, Andrew Mackay, being of sound mind, and with body resembling a ton of mashed banana packaged in Saran wrap, hereby swear that I shall abide by the following vows:

1: ONLY describe anything remotely scientific or mathematic in layman's terms for ease of use.

2: NEVER revisit already-written material and tamper, alter, or adjust anything. The account must remain honest and pure. If I do alter my two-week journey, it needs to be for good reason, and corroborated by *at least three* reputable sources.

3: NEVER use the word "diet." It has too many negative connotations, so I will use a substitute such as "adventure", "journey" etc.

4: I WILL weigh myself tomorrow, Monday, and not weigh myself again until the final day (Monday, July 8th - *Kebab Monday*). I do not want to measure my weight and become discouraged by potentially disappointing results. Better to just ignore it for now.

5: BE HONEST at all times. No part of this document shall be over-dramatized, fictionalized, or the subject of hyperbole. This extends to my inner thoughts and views.

I will also keep curse words to a minimum *and* PG-rated so as not to exclude sensitive or younger readers unnecessarily.

6: TELL NOBODY I am undertaking this task. I want to avoid the naysayers and anyone determined to put me off, *especially* if they mean well or display encouragement.

7: NO SEXUAL ACTIVITY until July 8th. *Kebab Monday.* You're obese, Mr. Mackay. You need to earn that orgasm, my friend.

***

And now, over to *you*, dear reader who isn't me. You need to make a vow, too. You vow NEVER to try *anything* I write about *unless* you a) read it right to the end, ***and*** b) seek guidance from your health care professional before you try.

If you read on and break the vow then I CANNOT be held responsible for what happens.

I'll take your continued reading of this book as confirmation and acceptance of this vow which absolves me of any and all responsibility in perpetuity.

***

And with that, ladies and gentlemen, boys and girls, I give you…

<u>THE HUNGER DIARIES</u>
Let's get to work…

Day 1, or:
"Getting' in Tuna"

"Make hunger thy sauce, as a medicine for health."
- Thomas Tusser

<u>*Monday, June 24th, 2019*</u>

Woke up at 11 am feeling completely normal and not hungry. Nothing new there - not physically, anyway. I'll admit that the only thing on my mind today is how much I *won't* be eating. *Eat less, move more*.

I have a plan as outlined in the introduction and I'm sticking to it.

As is usual for my mornings, I get dressed and switch on the radio player app on my phone. The usual dude (I won't name him) waffled on about Brexit and the state of our economy. I'm usually quite attentive mere seconds after I've woken from my slumber, but today, this radio presenter's voice is acting as background companionship as I approach the kitchen.

Kettle on. Computer on. And, for the first time in a long time, I pour myself a full glass of water. Down the hatch.

Gah, that tastes like nothing. Thank God for the sliver of apple squash (or Cordial) I've put in it otherwise it'd be intolerable. While I'm thinking of it, there appears to be an unspoken line with diluting juice. If you put the equivalent of an ant's tear in, you risk rendering the taste getting more awful - like there's something wrong with the kitchen sink. A murky solution that convinces you that the faucet is producing water right from Detroit this week. Pour *just* enough of the solution in and you're in the clear. It tastes of apples and less like zinc.

I think I've mastered the amount. I can't put a precise number on it - it's more of a gut feeling; my not insubstantial gut feeling, of course.

The kettle's boiled.

I grab my large mug and scoop out a tablespoon of perhaps the UK's most well-known brand of coffee. I want to avoid product placement, but it begins with an "N" and ends with an "E". No, it's not *noose* - I'll save that for when things don't go right and admit I'm a failure.

One and a half teaspoon of pure, ground coffee. Then, the sugar. Wait, hold on. Is this a good idea? Most people take one or two spoonfuls of sugar with their coffee. I've been pretty good at *not* doing this most of my life. Ask any of my friends and they'll tell you - "Huh? What do you mean exactly one fifth of a teaspoonful of sugar?" That's exactly what I mean. I guess it's a bit **Fool Yourself***, really*.

I slide the side of the extraordinarily small round bit of the spoon into the sugar bowl and lift up around twenty grains. I'm not kidding. I have a sixth sense when it comes to these things - that barrier I spoke about not a moment ago with the apple squash. *Just enough sugar for it to register on my tongue and convince myself I have more.*

Sip, sip, sip… yup, that's hit the spot. Pretty soon it'll be time for the first cigarette of the day, but first…

… I have to do what I do every morning. Check on my adverts for my books. I want to make sure they're performing, getting the clicks, and returning me a decent profit. Lately, I and other authors have noticed that ill-fated "June slump" rearing its head. This year is no different. My sales have dropped, and so have my page reads (we get paid a fraction of a penny per page you read if you have a Kindle Unlimited subscription.)

What's this got to do with my experiment? Well, I refer you to all the moments I've spoken about psychology. If I see I'm in the black - or, better, *the green* - in terms of profit, then it'll set the tone for my mood for the rest of the day. You would be the same, I'm sure.

I won't get any spurious and ill-advised attempts to raise the budget, or mess with the numbers, and risk losing even more money. So, I leave it alone. Yesterday's profits were borderline abysmal. Hopefully today will be an improvement. If only I was embarking on an experiment that could take my mind off it? Hmm.

Okay, that's me set up for a foul mood of a day. Time for a cigarette. The first one of the day serves two purposes for me:

1: It gets the initial nicotine hit blasting through my brain and waking me up right off the bat.

2: Perhaps most importantly, it encourages my bowels to perform - *and fast.*

As I look from my balcony at those who are making their way to the shopping mall from the industrial estate (yeah, my view really is that good!) I thank my lucky stars I work from home. I would never, ever contemplate leaving my apartment / hotel / friend's house without getting rid of it. When you get older this becomes an issue.

Toilet time - midday.

I am prepared for the fact that my stools are going to change, and possibly even the frequency (or lack thereof) of me actually moving my bowels. Last night I road-tested the tuna and apple thing for lunch, and then, for dinner, had my usual curry (Chicken Tikka Masala and rice, nan bread - all the good time!) but deliberately ate just a little bit less than I usually do. I guess I was mentally preparing for today.

And there lies the result in the toilet bowl. It looks like Jackson Pollack developed a fascination with my u-bend and only had dark brown paint to hand.

Who knows? If I take a picture of it and frame it, I could pretend it's genuine. There must be some lonely moron out there who'd buy it. (I didn't take a picture of it. Don't worry, there's no surprise on page 58 or anything).

As is usual for my fatter-than-fat lifestyle of processed food and endless trips to the kebab van, I'm not hungry in the morning. This morning is no different. I wonder if that will change over the course of the next two weeks?

A couple more cigarettes down, and I've done my work for today. All five minutes of it, if I'm brutally honest with myself.

Now, in the car, and off to my regular retreat to a nearby coffee store…

1 pm. Almost every day I'll break away from whatever I'm doing (or not) and visit a very well-known coffee franchise which I will rename *Bean There, Done That*. I'll grab a small, white Americano. In the US this would be known as a black filtered coffee. The "white" refers to creamer. I'll tear open a sugar packet and shake a few grains of regular white sugar in, stir it, and go outside to sit, smoke, listen to the radio, and watch the world go by.

If I'm honest, what I'm actually doing is watching the people drift by; male, female, sometimes both, short, tall, fat, thin, over-sized vertically (infrequent), over-sized horizontally (far more common), cute, ugly, over eighty, under five, and everyone else this particular shopping center attracts at lunchtime.

I have an idea. It'll seem strange, but in the long-term it might produce some interesting results.

I'll make sure that whenever someone looks my way, I'll smile back. It'd be interesting to see how they respond. Not much use while I'm sitting in front of the store window, though. It's a ridiculously warm day, and I've already chugged three cigarettes in a row. I'm still not hungry.

I've counted no fewer than fifty women who, under different personal circumstances, I would certainly *consider*, given half a chance.

The problem is that when you're fat, people tend to be less kind, less persuasive, and less receptive to ideas.

I walk back to my car and drive by the house we're hoping to move to next month. It's become something of a habit, now. The mission to complete has begun. I'm taking an alternate route home in the vague hope that someone up there is watching down on me and thinking "Aww, bless, look at him. Maybe we should speed this godforsaken nightmare up a bit for him" or something.

I get home around 1:45 pm with little desire to eat. Alas, it's time to have the first meal of the first day.

One can of drained tuna in brine. I add light "sneeze" of Cayenne powder and a whisper of black pepper. Doesn't look too bad. Doesn't smell too bad, either.

Then, there's the apple. It's called Granny Smiths, and it looks great - like a big, green ball of love. Cut into four quarters, and the spiny, black innards gouged out from the middle. Job done.

As the fork travels to my lips with the first delivery of dead, pink fish flesh, I make the decision to *eat slowly*. I dunno why, I just do it. I'm no scientist or dietitian, as you know, but my brain is telling me "eat slow, take your time, and your body will process it better." What basis I have for this fact? None at all.

The first bite is actually very nice. In fact, the whole darn thing is tasty. I got through the tin of tuna in about fifteen minutes whilst watching a YouTube video of Boris Johnson being shouted at by some protesters. Actually, now that I think about it, Boris himself lost a lot of weight earlier in the year. I suggest he did it because he knew there'd be a leadership contest coming up. It worked, whatever the reason. And have you seen that hot girl he's dating now? The one he dumped his wife for? You don't get quality like that unless you're extremely good-looking or incredibly rich. Huh, maybe the weight loss wasn't for her, then. Who knows. Who cares.

Now, to the apple. Not much to report. It tasted like an apple. But you know something funny? It crunched as I bit into it. The first time I've noticed because, let's face it, there aren't many bites to be had.

That's lunch.

3pm… I've consumed, by my calculations, two coffees, the equivalent of two tall glasses of apple squash, a tin of tuna, and an apple.

It's important to note that the data in calories at the end of this chapter is made up by me. I took what the packet recommended and added another ten. When it comes to the coffee (whole creamer and a sneeze of sugar) I am convinced that it comes to around fifty calories. My non-existent degree in mathematics tells me this is pure fiction. It's probably more in the 20 cal area.

But I like the challenge. The overcompensation. We'll see the grand total at the end of this day, but much of it will have been inflated - much like my waist, chin, and chest area over the years.

5pm. Went out for a walk around the shopping mall a stone's throw from my apartment. I'm quite hungry now. I've put it down to the water in apple and tuna. I dunno, there's just something about those two items that, in my mind, seems to bring about visions of waterfalls and oceans. Of course it would. Tuna is fish, after all. Duh. But *water* - the one thing that's making my stomach rumble.

Oh boy, it rumbled good. But that's okay. Only a couple hours till Amelia is home and I can have dinner.

But what if dinner isn't enough? What if I get hungry? To make matters worse, I'm walking past KFC and the stank is wafting out through the door.

I avoid KFC as my stomach growls again. This time, I'm sure a cashier in The brand fashion store - some sixteen thousand miles away - heard it. Time head back home and reconsider my life.

7:10 pm - I pick Amelia up in our car and we drive to a leading supermarket retailer whose name begins with "T" and with "O", with a sort of "esc" middle.

Our mission - fascina
wants to buy a sack of ja
Americans call, simply, "
had to buy last night in
fortnight of hell I'm pu
if not supportive, thou
suggested the Cayenn
and it worked.

I won't be mak
that I can tell yc
I eat m
potato
brain,
con

We bought some mo...
the fiber in my diet. Besides, every smoker kn...
cigarette tastes approximately 109.05% better after a
banana. Much like chocolate tastes after you have pure
orange juice, but with less ashy breath.

Forty-five minutes in the oven, and the potato itself is
ready. Looks okay to me.

"Do you want anything with it?"

"Nope."

I cut the thing into four quadrants and watch the
steam plume out, reminding me of just how hot this
bugger really is. And, me being me, I underestimate its
temperature when I shove the first clump in my mouth.

Jeez, the pain. Feels like my tongue has liquefied and
turned into a duvet made of molten lava.

A quick swig of squash will put the fire out, and
hopefully not leave some silly burn that'll take two days to
rectify.

g that mistake over and over again,

.nango-flavored yogurt straight after the
_g_ain, really slowly. A curious thing enters my
.ourtesy of **_Fool Yourself._** I somehow managed to
.ince myself that I hadn't eaten a potato. Instead, I'd
.aten a big, fat double cheeseburger with bacon. Ugh, just
typing that last sentence is making my mouth water!

But, it worked. I swear I could even taste some of the
animal fat in my mouth. It turns out I'm a really, really
good liar - especially to myself. And why wouldn't that be
the case? I've spent most of my thirties convincing myself
I'm "not that bad" in the weight department, usually
accompanied by a slight angling of my body in the mirror.

No, _I had that cheeseburger._ Suddenly, it felt like I'd eaten
it. The rest of the yogurt slunk down my throat and into
my stomach with relative ease.

It's a little after 8:30 pm, now, and I've thought that
having that one banana I'm allowed would go down well
around 11:30 pm - about two or three hours before bed
time.

Ha. Nice try.

I had the banana at 10 pm, an hour earlier than
advertised, because I _was really, really hungry!_ Wolfed it
down. My stomach rumbled up a storm prior to that. Most
normal people would think "Oh, I'm still hungry" - but
not me. No, I took that insane grumbling sound as my
stomach shrinking. Getting smaller. Contracting. Or

whatever it is that bodily organs do. Squelch Squelch… grumble… stomach shrinking. Surely there's some scientific fact in that assessment, right? Probably not, but who cares. It's what I think and feel (sort of) so that's that.

I end up watching some awful movie online and give up to conduct research on the conveyancing process. How much longer is this house-move going to take? It's been ten weeks already, and all the sites are telling me the norm is 8-12 weeks. Still no sign of completing.

Then, it suddenly hits me. I've started this ridiculous experiment for a few reasons, but one of them is to occupy my mind until our house completion goes through. We're selling our apartment and moving to a house nearby. We have a seller who's a cash buyer. It's a small, three-pronged chain. I'm getting impatient, now. Typical me.

Moving to this new house means I'll get that writing room and office I've always dreamed of, and can work in peace - even with Amelia at home. Don't get me wrong, she's very supportive and an absolute star. She wants me to do well. But… I can't write with other people in the room for some reason. Even now as I write this, she's gone to bed early. She sits on the sofa right behind my right shoulder.

I digress.

As you get older, time moves quicker. Months become weeks, and weeks become days. I remember when I was a kid, about six years old, waiting the entire summer vacation from school for *Ghostbusters* to arrive in theaters. It seemed like *years* away. Now, we have remakes and sequels of it almost every other week which, strictly speaking, is way off my original point. But whatever.

I write most of this chapter after the film finishes, brush my teeth and go to bed. Just as I switch off the computer, something incredibly frightening happens…

It's 3 am.

The room starts spinning as I stumble to the bedroom to disrobe. I just about manage to get my clothes off and walk, naked, to the bathroom. I barely make it. I feel as if I'm going to be sick. My shoulders, forehead and back start sweating.

I'm afraid of actually blacking out entirely.

But… and this is typical me, too… I squeeze the toothpaste out of the tube and think "If I die, then I die." I also think "At least toothpaste has a taste, and it'll be yummy."

I brush my teeth and find I'm right. The nausea subsides enough for me to gargle some mouthwash.

When I climb into bed, usually I'll read a few news stories on my phone until I feel my eyelids get heavy. This time, I'm just glad to be lying down.

Glad that this didn't happen while I was out shopping.

Very glad it didn't happen while I was driving.

In bed, I closed my eyes, exhaled… and then everything went black.

<u>Calories Consumed:</u>

Tuna = 120

Apple = 80

Jacket Potato = 250

Yogurt = 55

Banana = 100

Half a handful of cashew nuts: 100

3 x Coffee = 150

3 x Squash = 60

Grand Total: 915

Day 2, or:
"Full Metal Jacket Potato"

"I aimed at the public's heart, and by accident I hit it in the stomach."
- Upton Sinclair

<u>*Monday, June 25th, 2019*</u>

I am writing this chapter at 12:20 am - twenty minutes after the day closed. Amelia went to bed about an hour ago, which is great, because it means I can tap-tap-tappity-tap on my keyboard to my heart's content with my classical music mix on YouTube playing in the background.

Why do you care? Let me explain.

She sent me a text 34 minutes ago while she was in bed drifting off. I always have my phone in silent, so I didn't hear it when it first came in. So, when I saw it (34 minutes post-send) I ran into the bedroom and asked what was up. She said she'd sent me a link to a news story.

We're moving from the city center to a place in Chrome Valley (*hmm*, where did I get that name from? Check out my other books and find out!) which is much quieter. It's a leafy suburb mostly populated by retired citizens and is comparatively peaceful. I should know; I've stalked the damn place often enough during this long process of trying to get moved.

The news story reveals that Chrome Valley had its first robbery a mere three streets away from where we're going to be moving to. I rather thought that the area was safe. No crimes had been reported for months or years; and I should know, I've researched the crime figures obsessively enough. What a downer.

Does it affect my experiment? Not remotely. It's a bit of a side-track, granted, but I want you to feel as if you're really here with me and getting an idea of my mental processes.

Why?

Well, during day two, I learned about some of the side effects of this stupid endeavor. Namely, I'm forgetting things. I'm not lightheaded nor sick, nor am I especially hungry (more on that later) but I did commit a few acts of retardation during my second day of dietary fun and games. And by *retardation*, I really do mean that in the literal, dictionary sense; slow and somewhat backwards in my actions.

Okay, let's recount. I got up at 11 am and forgot to switch on the radio. I'll admit, I thought the morning sounded a little different today. No Mister Man on the talk radio app spouting off about Brexit and how evil and vile (duo anagram - yippee!) Boris Johnson is. I'm sorry to keep bringing this up, but it's my life, you understand. I'm a glutton (though hopefully not for much longer, food-wise) for punishment. Maybe I just feel superior to the dude I'm listening to when I have my morning coffee.

But not before I do my new morning ritual of hydration. One full glass of water with a whisper of apple squash. Gulped it down in one. Now, I feel bloated, as if I've eaten an entire Thanksgiving turkey. Kettle goes on.

I do my five-minute work for the day. Check those ads. Oh my! I reduce my daily budget drastically and suddenly I'm making more money. Eh? How does that work? Well… *if it ain't broke, don't fix it* - as they say.

I up my budget 300% because I'm stupid. I'll guess we'll see just how dumb that move was tomorrow morning.

Coffee, hint of sugar, hint of whole fat milk. I sip my morning beverage during my ad work and then peruse two websites for my daily injection of news-based nonsense. I've perfected the art of being in-the-know and up-to-date with events by checking an extremely far left news site and counterbalancing it by reading an even more extreme far right one. That's what I call balance. It hasn't gone unnoticed by me that the ladies are much prettier in the latter's publication.

Um, *where was I?*

Oh yeah. The first cigarette of the day finished, and I'm not hungry in the slightest. I wonder how the re-emergence of a potato and a tin of tuna will go down. I suppose I mean that literally. Let's go to the bathroom and see…

That's interesting. I had expected some semblance of constipation with this diet. Surprisingly, the stool flowed out just fine. I check my phone. It's just after midday and I do my usual surface check of Facebook to make sure I wish those I care about a happy birthday, and see what rubbish everyone's talking about. I find that's *plenty* of time for Facebook for one day. Combining it with my daily bowel movement seems somewhat fitting.

I gave up on social media about a year ago. It's just not worth it anymore. With the extra time I've gained much more done. Perhaps I'll tell you about it someday.

So, this morning's bowel movement was just fine. More turgid and "healthy" I guess is the word I'd use, here, and not the 3D version of the opening scene of *Saving Private Ryan* with feces standing in for all the blood. Nice.

Before I toodle off for my daily jaunt to *Bean There, Done That*, I notice something strange. Despite not being hungry *whatsoever* my mouth is watering up a storm. Quite a lot, and quite often. I find I'm spitting long, clear ropes of saliva into my balcony ashtray; every ten seconds or so, in between puffs on my cigarette.

This would go on all day. It's still happening now as I write this sentence. In fact, just bringing it up in the last paragraph is drawing attention to the fact I'm salivating. Only, I can't spit it onto the keyboard. I'm having to swallow it. It's not exactly swallowing, more a trickle down the back of my tongue and into my throat.

And now, writing *that* last paragraph is making it worse. Ugh. Why do I never stop salivating? What if I keep ingesting my own spit? Hang on, how many calories are there in saliva, anyway? Oh god, it's all going wrong.

You may remember earlier in this chapter that I mentioned… something. Hang on, let me scroll back up and check.

Oh yeah. *Forgetfulness.*

(Ba-dum Tch!)

I have mild OCD (Obsessive Compulsive Disorder.) Not in that crappy "Oh yeah, I hate it when my CD collection isn't in alphabetical order" kind of a way - I mean serious OCD. I don't switch lights on and off when I enter a room. I don't ruthlessly wash my hands five times or anything. Nah, my OCD is peculiar. It's mostly to do with symmetry and shapes.

For example, if you were to take a look at my work desk you'll see that it's clutter-that-isn't-clutter. My papers (both work-related and moving-house-related) are perfectly aligned with the corner of the table. My laptop is perfectly perpendicular to the little desk behind it. Even my pack of smokes is perfectly square just beside it. As I type, my keyboard is exactly centered in front of the screen - and make no mistake - I *will* stop typing just to readjust it.

What does this kind of psychology mean for a diet? Who knows. A sneak preview of the answer surely lies in not referring to this daft process as a *diet* - but an experiment. The word diet has all sorts of connotations with it.

Let's you, dear reader, and I ponder on this together for a moment. When you hear or read the word *diet*, what do you automatically think of? I'll tell you what I think of. I picture a man with a huge stomach and manboobs getting squeezed around the waist by a massive cartoon hand so hard that his head bulges and his tongue kites out of his massive red lips.

Write to me and let me know what you think of. I'm curious.

Aaaaaaanyway… my OCD sees me do a few very helpful things. If I need to do something the following day, (e.g. a shopping list, or take my secure card key to the bank) I'll put it in my shoe. That way when I put my shoes on - and who doesn't? - hey presto! An instant reminder, and just before I leave the house. I even put our car's heavy duty carrier bag for shopping ON TOP of my shoes to remind me to take it to the car when the next time I go.

Today - and don't ask me how - I left my apartment *without* my earphones. Yeah, you heard me right. I walked out without them and I *never* do that. Ever.

I even closed the door and locked it before remembering that my breast pocket felt a bit weird. Like something was missing.

I walked back in and grabbed them, and then wondered if I hadn't gone completely mad.

1 pm, and I'm sitting outside *Bean There, Done That* with my small, white Americano and umpteen cigarettes, watching the world go by. And, quite honestly, a flurry of beauties. Today is really, really, really warm. Like thirty-two degrees Celsius (89F), or something, and the British humidity is ridiculously violent. Parts of me I didn't know I had are sweating like a blind vegan in an abattoir. It's warm and this week is only going to get hotter.

I'm still not hungry. It's been fifteen hours since I last ate the banana at 10 pm last night. My stomach isn't growling and, curiously, I'm not spitting right now - although that could be because I'm drinking coffee and smoking.

As I sip on my coffee I wonder - briefly - how this silly project of mine is going to play out. I mean, how long can I really sustain (significantly) less than 1000 calories per day? I suppose the fact you're reading this, if it ever escapes from my computer, means I didn't die.

Or did I?

Maybe my fellow author friends clambered together to complete the diary and expatiate on how stupid I was for doing it.

I'm not dead, yet, and that's progress as far as I'm concerned. Let's put it another way. If I don't shed a fair amount of body weight in fourteen days with this diet, then I won't have reprogrammed my appetite so I can eat sensibly from this point forward. And, if I don't do that, I'll still be obese, and that will kill me eventually. So, my theory is thus:

45

Prevent yourself from dying of obese-related illnesses - or die trying.

Why prolong the misery? Most of the causes of death are due to shoddy diets. A close second is smoking. I don't especially care if I die early but I *do* know others who care. At least, I think they care. No, silly me. Of course they do. Now I'm rambling.

Lunch.

Tuna, Cayenne and black pepper sprinkles (honestly, this tiny addition is terrific!) and four slices of apple. You already know the calorie intake for this, but I'll recap it at the end of the day for the sake of document.

I wasn't even hungry for lunch if I'm honest. I had to go out to run some errands. I mention this because I *briefly* entertained the notion of skipping lunch altogether like some insane madman. About 3.5 seconds after the thought crashed into my cranium, I immediately decided against it.

See, this is the thing when you're undertaking a ~~diet~~ project. Or keeping a journal, which is another great motivator. You start thinking weird stuff. Every mouthful of whatever good food you've committed yourself to becomes the enemy. Biting into an apple? You may as well have swallowed an entire lamb kebab smothered in mayonnaise and lard. See that first mouthful of tuna? That was 16,088,577 empty calories, you fat so-and-so. Look at you and your stupid bloated stomach being all "Oooh, look at me, I eat food!" and stuff. Ugh.

I'm sorry but it's true. Hell, just last week I was eating a lamb kebab drenched in chili and garlic sauce with hardly any salad with it. And a large chips with salt and vinegar. I had absolutely *no* notion of going on a diet. The day before I had a chicken chow mein (noodles), egg fried rice, crispy chili beef and a bag of prawn crackers. And that was just *dinner*.

As I write this chapter - and in particular that last sentence - my mouth is watering. I realize this is only the second day of the experiment, but I simply cannot believe I was doing that to my body. It goes to show that eating and food - the whole ugly business of sustenance and *not dying from starvation* - is purely habitual and psychological. It really is.

Ask me again in a week if I feel the same way. Who knows? It could be that this time next week I'll have developed a wasting disease, or some heretofore unknown wasting condition that eats the muscles in my hands and I won't be able to type. In that event, I'll using dictation software (if my wife helps me set it up because I have no muscles in my forearms).

I hit the shopping mall around 3:30 pm - in other words, four hours before dinner. Yesterday, all I could think about was food. How long it had been since I ate and when I'd eat again. Today, that notion all but disappeared.

And another bizarre thing happened that I want to record if I ever have to revisit this diary.

As I exited my apartment block, I convinced myself I was already at my target weight. I'm not joking, by the way. The strings on my linen trousers had loosened (but that could just be down to me being abnormally well-endowed) and I had to hitch them up again (no, seriously, leave it okay? People who've been with me call me *the legend*) and re-tie them in private (FFS, leave it alone, okay? How do you think this fat monstrosity of whale blubber got a beautiful wife in the first place? It's not because of my charming personality, I can tell you.) (Okay, maybe it was, but that's not the point.) (Seriously, just leave it, okay.)

Amelia and I met in our early-to-mid-twenties when I was, shall we say, *leaner* (and therefore, unrealistically gifted in the pants department - whereas now I'm modestly *Olympic*) - and she was more, shall we say, less discerning about a potential lifelong suitor.

The point is that I began behaving and walking like I was thin. Can you imagine? There's me, your humble narrator / writer / thing walking with his shoulders back and head held high like he was Christian Bale in *The Machinist*. It felt good. The warm weather didn't bother me. Who cared if I was sweating, anyway? It just meant that I had an excuse to strip naked and get in the shower and admire my beautiful, well-toned body. At least, that's what I saw.

What others saw, no doubt, was a double-chinned, arrogant fatso waddling up the pathway thinking he was God's gift to... *God knows*. That awkwardly-shaped, middle-aged never-was, has-been striding so confidently toward the shopping mall - no doubt headed for KFC or burger stand to fill his fat, ugly face with burgers and chicken and biscuits and gravy until he got so fat that if he dared to jump in the air he'd get stuck. Not that he could jump, anyway, given his recent Body Mass Index result. The misguided and obese cretin would probably break his ankles just trying it.

Ah, whatever. It's all about the **Fool Yourself** methodology, as I've mentioned in the introduction. It's alive and well, here. I really need to patent it.

Now, onto the interesting bit. Despite my enactment of *Shallow Hal* (or should I say in spite of it?) my confidence meant that I was acting out of character. I smiled at people - male and female - as I walk past them. Some of them smiled back. One or two of them even a bit flirtatiously. And as for the *women...*

I think the point I'm trying to make is that if you *think and act* thin, you may as well be thin. Of course, that only works for you internally. On the outside, you may still be a big, fat bucket of pig sick but you're engaging with others and they engage back. They smile. They acknowledge you. Maybe Jehovah's Witnesses and the homeless can learn something from this? Perhaps they already have. Maybe I'm late to the party. Maybe I'm talking garbage. Maybe, just maybe, I've made my point and can't think of a prophetic way to end this paragraph.

I ran my errands like the over-sized lump of fat-on-legs I really am and made my way back home.

I met my wife at the station and we went for a coffee. Well, she got some weird, unpronounceable cold thing ending in "cino" and I had my usual small, white Americano with a dust of sugar. That's three coffees I've had today and, around five hours after lunch, it was quite tasty. I have a feeling my taste buds are going to get a reboot by the time this is done.

Also, I spent most of the afternoon with one bullet of sugar-free chewing gum in my mouth. I usually only chew when I go to the movies. I usually go on weekends. Because I smoke, I need to chew throughout the movie - or, at least, I *think* I need to chew. Perhaps I don't? As I'm writing this I can see a sequel to this book rearing its head. Maybe on giving up smoking? I don't know. One goal at a time and all that.

One thing I can say with all certainty is that being a smoker really helps. It's well known that cigarettes contain carcinogens and will ultimately kick your ass six feet under quicker than the government and its high-octane, austerity-riddled existence we're all experiencing could ever hope to. We also know it's a very effective appetite suppressor. It's true - it does suppress the appetite. I'm no psychologist as you know, but it must be something to do with the act of putting something in your mouth. Maybe I should take up fellatio and give my lungs a break.

Amelia and I got home. She complained about the humidity of the day. She has to take the train to work every day, but thankfully it's air conditioned. To be fair, I think everyone's spouse made the same comment today at some point during the day. The humidity was slapping sweat under my "titch bits" and I can't imagine how uncomfortable it must have been for those with bigger boobs than mine. *Humidititties*? I like that word. I must use it somewhere, soon. Oh, I already did.

Dinner time came around 8 pm - and on tonight's menu we have a jacket potato with absolutely nothing added, followed by a light yogurt. Yum.

And I'm not being sarcastic. 45 minutes in the oven, and the potato was delicious. The skin was even better. It felt like heaven. Ask me this time next week how I feel about a potato for dinner. Here's the weird thing. I wasn't even hungry. Can you believe that?

The moment my nostrils caught the waft of them being cooked I got a little bit hungry. We cooked all ten of them in one go so we wouldn't have to wait 45 minutes each night to eat. I say "we" - Amelia isn't doing the project with me. We agreed I'd do road test it first, figure out the exact point at which I died, and she could dial it back by two days - and hopefully lost a few pounds in the process before my life insurance pays out.

She had one potato just like I did. She followed it up with some other stuff like crisps and chocolate - I don't know for sure that she ate because the sofa is behind my desk. I found myself *not* craving what she was having. I usually polish off a large dinner with a huge chocolate bar, sometimes two. But today I didn't. And I didn't do it yesterday, either.

My main goal is to hit 12 stone, and a part of that process was to shrink my appetite. I figured it'd take three days to do it (shrink my appetite, not reach 12 stone!) and I've reached the end of the second day.

My stomach didn't growl but I am still salivating, although it seems to have stopped now. My mouth is dry. Maybe I'll keep it that way till I go to sleep.

The best thing, now? I'm not hungry and it's nearly 2 am. I have half a glass of apple squash-laced water on my desk. I might even skip the cashew nuts.

I don't need them.

Calories Consumed:

Tuna = 120

Apple = 80c

Jacket Potato = 250

Yogurt = 55

Banana = 100

3 x Coffee = 150

3 x Squash = 60

1 x Chewing Gum = 5c

Grand Total: 820

Day 3, or:
"Unlucky Number 8"

"I'm not beautiful, okay, and I never will be.
And I'm fine with that. But when you go around saying I'm
something that I'm not, it's just… it's just not nice."
- Rosemary, *Shallow Hal (2001)*

<u>*Wednesday, June 26th, 2019*</u>

I didn't get that insufferable feeling of nausea I experienced when I crawled into bed last night. Thank God for that. I was hoping it wouldn't be a recurring pre-bedtime effect of this silly experiment. If that had been the case then I might have quit already. I never want to feel that way again. I stress the word *want*, here, of course; I'm fully prepared for the fact that it might happen again. If it does then I just hope it's somewhere safe - and preferably with a bed nearby.

I woke up at 11 am once again today and for the first time in a long time I felt hungry. My stomach ceased to growl (or shrink, as my mind thinks of it) now, but the salivation is still happening. The hunger wasn't annoying, but it was unexpected. As I mentioned in a previous entry I am never hungry when I wake up. Back in my teaching days, I'd often survive on coffee and cigarettes until dinner. Of course, dinner would inevitably be something fried; cheeseburgers, kebabs, slices of lard, that kind of thing.

Amelia and I won't be keeping Gordon Ramsey awake at night any time soon. Neither of us can cook; she's too busy and I am, frankly, something of a Luddite when it comes to handling anything other than my [removed on editorial advice]. I could screw up beans on toast. Ask me to cut a sandwich and it'll look like I had a stabbing contest with a loaf of bread.

Another good thing about being married is that my wife can work the oven. Use the washing machine. I can't. I mean, I could learn, but I haven't because *reasons*.

So, naturally, much of what we used to eat is processed food and takeout. We bought sandwiches from the supermarket rather than a loaf of bread and fillings. Amelia and I are exceptionally lazy in some respects and ruthlessly efficient in others. Food is both our weaknesses. Amelia will think nothing of snacking before dinner time and still manage to not gain much weight.

I've always had a problem with weight. I was a chubby kid right the way from birth (despite weighing just 5 lbs as a baby) to the end of high school. When I hit college (which I guess our American readers will recognize as the last two years of high school) I went on a ruthless regime of cold, non-processed food. Mostly sandwiches and apple squash. I remember it vividly. It was the Spring of 1996, my first year of college, and for about five months all I ate was ham sandwiches with a sliver of butter. The pounds melted away and I became thin. A year later I gained a fair bit of weight, but not nearly to the whale-like level I was before. That was my last attempt at a serious diet, but over the years - in my twenties, thirties - the weight slowly piled back on... and then off again... and crept back in. A yo-yo effect to a fault us fatties have all experienced, I'm sure.

At least I've been through an extreme diet once before, albeit twenty-three years ago when I was something of a spring chicken. I didn't have back problems back then - when losing weight actually meant something. If I hadn't gone through the sandwich diet I'd have ended up around 350 lbs (over 20 stone) for most of my adult life and, it's fair to say, a lot of the luck I've had in life might not have happened.

Take, for example, the first moment I laid eyes on Amelia outside my college back in September of 2004. That almost certainly would have played out differently. A vision of beauty from a faraway place, in my eyes. In her eyes? A fat, sweating mound of mashed potatoes in a black shirt, blinking its eyelids at her in what would surely be received as some kind of gargantuan, perverted fetish. We wouldn't have gone on to have our first date at *Thai Heaven* (the restaurant around the corner), nor go on to get married. I dread to think that there's an alternate universe out there where Amelia lays eyes on a 1,589,601 lb Andrew and immediately turns away, ostensibly in disgust, but then to projectile vomit over the wall in abject horror.

Let's face facts. No one likes a fatty, do they? Oh, sure, we all say we do in polite society. Even us fatties hate other fatties. I'm convinced of it. I'll no doubt talk about my views on fat shaming in a later chapter (it's not for now as I have some events to recount for today) save to say that I think fat shaming is a bit of a stupid term. I don't want anyone *shamed* because of their weight. What I *do* want is to draw attention to their health and how they might set about fixing it.

I remember thinking to myself as I stood on my balcony and had the first coffee of the day that I wished I had more friends. Don't get me wrong, I do have *some* friends. None of them are close - either geographically or personally. In that respect they're not much use to me in terms of this project I'm undertaking. Now that I'm a best-selling author, I mostly spend all my time alone and writing. I converse with other authors through Skype and chat, but it's not physical contact. And that's what I need. I *want* someone I trust to say "Hey, you fat pig, keep it going," or "A diet, you say? Ha, yeah. I'll believe it when I see it!" What I do not want is someone I know to smirk and say, "Meh. That'll never work."

I know it's only been three days, but already I'm discovering that I absolutely *love* being told I can't do something. You know why I love it? Because it makes me mad and want it all the more. If someone told me that I couldn't tear the (white, lacy) panties off Jennifer Lawrence on the first night because a) I'm not her type, or because b) I'm too fat, then I'll rise to that challenge. Particularly *this* one. If there was a *serious* chance I might get her in bed, just give me six months. I'll make damn sure all that fat is gone. I'll make *damner* sure that the last remnants of fat in my pelvic area will burn off with her for sixteen hours straight.

I jest, but you get my point. Actually, my *two* points. Determination, and no one likes fat people.

I finish my coffee and wonder why my bowels aren't shifting. Of course, it's because I haven't have the first cigarette of the day. Three-and-a-half minutes later, and yet *another* five minutes shaved off my life due to my nicotine intake, I feel the urge to go and lose weight courtesy of the toilet bowl.

Just walking towards the bathroom I know this particular bowel movement isn't going to be an award-winner. I figure it'll be small and easy to remove - and thus, it was.

When I take a dump I check Facebook, as I've mentioned before. I passed this morning's stool in about three seconds. I actually used less paper to wipe (sorry, TMI? Well, if you're stupid enough to replicate what I am doing, let this be a warning!) and all was done. I didn't even have time to check my daily dose of socialites complaining and whining about how bad a day they're having already? Wow. An entire day without Facebook whatsoever. Bliss.

All I hoped by this point was that my bowel movements would be *regular*. Full marks on that front. At approximately midday, now, we're on form. I hope that's true of tomorrow morning, too.

Before I braved my two-mile drive to *Bean There, Done That*, I find myself on the balcony smoking another cigarette. Halfway through a puff, my saliva builds up as I inhale. So I spit it towards the ashtray on the floor - and miss entirely. A long, gelatinous rope of spit slaps against the glass panel and slinks towards the ground.

Why? Because today is incredibly windy, and a lot cooler than expected. The wind is *fierce* by all accounts - particularly when you're on a balcony five floors up in one of Chrome Valley's tallest structures. Yes, I'm still salivating, perhaps a little more right now because I'm feeling hungry. I guess I should take that to mean I am human.

12:30 pm, *Bean There, Done That*. My usual spot outside the storefront at my favorite table. All of them were empty, which is unusual for the office lunch rush. I stop the pretty little vixen who serves my coffee and ask her to use semi-skimmed milk instead of full-fat from now on - which she duly applies to the piping hot mixture.

I suck on my first cigarette whilst listening to my morning dose of anti-Brexit complaining from one of the UK's foremost and outspoken authorities on the matter. And now he's talking about what happened at Prime Minister's Questions. I don't particularly care at this point in time. If you had caught me last week, or this time last month, I'd have soaked up everything he was saying.

Today, though, the voice is sort of drifting into my ear and acting as a background noise - again. I get *really* comfortable in my chair and cross my right leg over my left, and lean my cheek on my fist like some bizarre Rodin sculpture. Then, I feel my eyes close and - more weirdly - the side of my head rests gently against the giant glass window on the storefront.

I begin to drift away with half a lit cigarette in my left hand and - BAM! - come-to immediately. That has never happened in my life. Falling asleep at the table, for that is what I did. No one saw it, though.

I feel a stinging sensation on my thumb and look down to find it's bleeding. WTF? How did that happen? Then, that zinc-like taste we all know and love forms in my mouth. My upper-right incisor had sunk into the fleshy part of my thumb. Even as I type this sentence I can feel it, but it doesn't hurt any more. This is ridiculous, I remember thinking at the time. Am I *so* hungry now that I've turned to self-cannibalism? I must have done it without thinking of it. And, now, the relentless saliva build-up is flooding back. Another cigarette and a huge gulp of coffee should take care of that - and it does.

When you go to *Bean There, Done That* at approximately the same time every day without fail, you tend to see the same patrons come and go. There are a few I see all the time. I've never spoken to any of them so I don't know their names. Quite honestly, I couldn't care less. But they're the closest thing I have to regular friends (!)

Let me give you a quick rundown of the regular players, because I find it amusing - and relevant to the diary.

1: *Unlucky Number 8*. Named because when you look at her standing up, her top and bottom resemble a figure eight. How to put it nicely? Hmm. She's a hideously obese girl in her early twenties. She wears spectacles. Sometimes, I sneakily eavesdrop on her conversations on the phone. She's truly ugly inside and out, and that's not a criticism.

I've deduced from my private investigations into her calls that she's unemployed and spends her time out of the house so her father doesn't shout at her for being a morbidly obese waste of time. So, she comes to *Bean There, Done That* with her laptop and phone under the pretense of searching for gainful employment. She never conducts research on available jobs, though, as far as I can see. Instead, she spends her time chatting to her little friends about how she hates everything and her life and how she doesn't care if she dies. If only her father knew she spends her time messing around on Instagram and talking to her friends about boys instead of looking for work. Maybe one day I'll follow her home and find out where she lives and post a note through the door with evidence. Maybe I won't.

2: *Love Roller Coaster.* A spindly, withered lady in her seventies. She's in a wheelchair (bless her) and moves at approximately 0.00000178 millimeters per hour. Sometimes she rolls past and doesn't visit the store. Sometimes she does. And when she does, she needs help from some kind-hearted Samaritan to hold the door open for her. I've *never* held the door open for her, as it happens. Someone usually beats me to it.

3: *Golden Oldie.* A quite attractive lady in her sixties who smokes like a trouper. She looks a little like Pia Zadora and she usually sits opposite me. She's cute in a mommy-type-of-way. She's never looked at me once.

4: *Stick Thin.* In his fifties, this dude walks with a stick and is very thin indeed. He walks like John Wayne, if John Wayne and been kicked in the nuts by the T-800 from *The*

Terminator. I'm not sure which came first - the extreme weightlessness or the need for a stick, but either way, it's unfortunate and not a good look. He could very well be ill, but I don't know. I'm not sure who the woman with him is. It could be his wife or mother. Hard to tell. I'm guessing the former.

5: *Stander.* One of my favorites of the regular punters. Instead of sitting at a table to smoke and drink, he *stands* at the table and scrolls through his cell phone whilst chain-smoking. He's short and stumpy and has been known to stand there for hours. In my messed-up mind, his record might be 4,598 hours straight without a bathroom break.

6: *Goddamn Weird Freak.* Dressed like Keanu Reeves in *The Matrix* no matter the weather, this freak of nature always, *always* turns up at 12:30, gets his drink, and then walks away in the direction of the car park. I once stood behind him in the line at the counter and caught him playing with a ladybug on his hand. Anyone would have puked at the sight, but not this dude - he just turned his hand around and let the critter climb all over fingers as if it was an everyday occurrence. I've no evidence to substantiate the claim I'm about to make, but I firmly believe that Goddamn Weird Freak has committed an act of atrocity so severe and repugnant that he should be in jail. A bit like when you look at our former Prime Minster David Cameron's face - you have no evidence, but you *just know* he's done something heinous, possibly along the lines of the holocaust.

All six of these individuals have appeared one way or another in the past three days - especially numbers 1, 4, and 6. I dunno about you, but I find people utterly fascinating. People-watching is great for authors. You cook up some great characters and "what ifs" for your stories. I bring this up because I am now on day three of this obstacle course and find myself looking mainly at two types of people:

1: Ridiculously beautiful women, and,

2: Ridiculously overweight men

I guess that tells you everything you need to know about my sexuality - not that it's any of your business.

There is no shortage of either of those two subsets of individual; a constant influx of both types stroll past every five seconds or so. It's hard to know where to look, or even start.

Today I counted at least fifty overweight men of various ages - mostly consigned to the twenties / thirties bracket. Some had ridiculous flabby breasts that tried to keep up with the bounce of their over-sized bellies. A former friend of mine a few years ago once told me something I've failed to forget, as you'll see with this next sentence of verbatim dialog:

"Andrew, now that my girlfriend is six months pregnant, all I'm doing is checking out beautiful women and desperately wanting to impregnate as many of them as I can."

Amelia and I don't have children, but as a red-blooded, (mostly) cis-gendered (heterosexual) attack helicopter, I figure there must be some truth in what my friend said. Because - check this out - all high-and-mighty extreme dieter Andrew Mackay sitting at this table chugging his third cigarette has news for you, the overweight rhino who's walking past - I'm doing a diet, and I want you to do it with me!

What? What do you mean you don't wanna do it? It's great! It's called The Hunger Diaries. Lose weight, write a diary. One encourages the other! No, you fool, it's not a diet - it's a game. Look, mate, you'll feel a lot better if you lost some weight and--

—Whoa! Hold up, Mackay. Who are you, of all people, to foist your not-unsubstantial gut onto others? Yeah, just because *you* are doing this diet doesn't mean you have to bore everyone else with it. Shut the hell up.

Okay, fine, I'll go home and have my insanely low-calorie lunch now.

Lunch rocks up at around 1:15 pm today. Guess what I had? Yep, a tin of tuna and an apple sliced into four parts.

I ate it the same way I ate it the previous two days - slowly. I washed it down with a glass of water, and all was well. Except I was still hungry.

Yesterday I noticed that I was forgetting things. Today is different. I'm remembering things just fine (perhaps because of the earphones incident yesterday) but today I'm noticing that I am slowing down.

Like *real, real slow…*

When I stand up and wash the plate I noticed I've done it slower. I've caught myself on a number of occasions - going to the balcony for a smoke, or the bathroom to pee - that I slow down and even stop and *think* ahead to make sure it's what I want to do and how I'll do it. That's pretty weird, huh? As a matter of fact, *everything* has ground to a near-halt; my reactions, my thoughts, my general being. I was razor-sharp driving home from the coffee place. Even as I type this at midnight on the day in question, the words are flowing like Hemingway. I'm talking about the *flow* and not the quality, obviously; I'm far superior to Hemingway in almost every respect, *and* I'm still alive. And don't get me started on my modesty, either.

I felt like taking a nap during the afternoon but I decided against it. I can't even remember the reason. I think it was something to do with my laptop needing updated and attended to, which took me all afternoon because I'm so slow…

7:10 pm. I pick Amelia up from the station in the car, and we end up at (drum roll) *Bean There, Done That* once again. Second time today for me. It's not *all that* unusual for me to visit twice in one day.

We sit outside at the other table by the window. I spark up a cigarette and tell her how everything is going. I *always* ask Amelia how her day was. Every day, without fail. She tells me what went down at work (she's not especially overjoyed with what happened) and then she asks me how my day was with a specific focus on the project at hand. I told her it was fine. I also told her that my writing a journal about this adventure was a good idea, because one begets the other.

I've even made a little mathematic equation for it: *Weight loss adventure + Journal = Two Birds Killed With One Stone* (which, coincidentally, is the amount of weight I am hoping to shed by "Kebab Monday", July 8th.) Put simply, writing for an hour or so every day is perpetuating this stupid project. If I quit the book, the weight loss adventure could be over. And if I quit the journey, there's not much of a book. My thinking is this; if you found *The Hunger Diaries* available for purchase at Amazon then you know I didn't quit.

We enter the supermarket and stock up on tins of tuna and more bananas and more apple squash. I find I'm going through the bottle of squash (Cordial) quicker than expected. We have vowed not to overstock food items because, hopefully, any day now we'll get a call from my solicitor telling me that we're going to move house.

Just another reason the waiting game is so unbearable, quite honestly. Buying in smaller amounts is annoying.

You may remember from yesterday's entry that Amelia and I batch-baked a bunch of jacket potatoes. This meant that preparing dinner only took five minutes in the microwave. Amelia forewarned me that this meant that tonight's potato wouldn't be as crispy or scrumptious as Tuesday's - and she was right.

The skin was soggy and damp. It tasted the same, but was missing that angelic halo of yellow loveliness from the night before. I ate it slowly, and waited half an hour to eat my mango yogurt. In that time I sat beside her on the sofa and massaged her legs.

My real agenda was for her to kiss me, or at least touch my face, to see if she noticed any difference. As I half-expected, she said "no" to my question "have you noticed anything different?" She said "no" with an ebullience usually reserved for doctors pushing bad news to their patients.

Here's the thing. Today I noticed that most of my wobbly parts were wobbling a bit less than usual. I think the word I'm searching for is *tighter*. I can *feel* something tightening in places.

First off, I am sure my chin is tighter. As I walk around in my unfashionable, but extremely comfortable, baggy clothes, I feel my inner thighs not rubbing together as much as they used to. I've never been especially fat on my arms. I don't have flabby bingo wings. My chest isn't bouncing as much and I think the weight in my stomach is dissipating.

The key word in all this is *think*. The **Fool Yourself** thing in full swing. Amelia assures me I'm still the fat bucket of pig feces I truly am (in other words, she said "No, I can't see any difference") but, damn it, stuff's gotten tighter since Monday. I dunno, perhaps it's all in the mind? Isn't everything?

I've decided I'll do a couple of things from tomorrow onward.

1: I won't eat the banana until two hours after I finish dinner (i.e. the follow-up yogurt.)

2: I might skip lunch altogether tomorrow just to see how my body responds. If I'm hungry come lunchtime, then I'll have the tuna and apple.

3: Exercise. Rather than drive the 2 miles to *Bean There, Done That*, I think I should walk it. Why not? The weather is nice.

A part of me (presumably the obese part) is really, really keen to see how I get on with just one potato and a yogurt. Half the calorie intake as (extremely unwisely) self-directed. The other part of me wants to *not die*. So, we'll see how that stupid second idea goes down.

The intention of this crash diet is to reduce my appetite, as you know. I figured three days would do it, and it appears to have worked - unless I've died in my sleep tonight, in which case it *worked a goddamn treat*. But, failing an early demise, I'm starting to think forward to Monday July 8th - the day after the two-week-long project of stupidity I'm putting myself through. What can I reasonably hope to sustain? I think a 1,200 calorie diet of vegetables and sensible food would be fine.

But I do know one thing.

I told Amelia that "Kebab Monday" would be my last entry into the journal. And on that day, dinner is going to be a giant, fat sweaty lamb kebab drenched in chili and garlic sauce and a side order of large chips with salt.

"Why on Earth would you do that?"

"Because I want to know if I feel any differently towards a food I adore."

True, that. Twelve days from now I'll go to that kebab van and come home and attempt to eat it. Will I gorge it all down? Will it taste any different? I dunno, but it's a goal, and (I hope) a fitting end to this book…

Calories Consumed:

Tuna = 120

Apple = 80c

Jacket Potato = 250

Yogurt = 55

Banana = 100

3 x Coffee = 150

4 x Squash = 80

Grand Total: 840

Day 4, or:
"The Pork Sword Strikes Back"

"Pork chops and bacon. My two favorite animals."
- Homer Simpson, *The Simpsons*

<u>*Thursday, June 27th, 2019*</u>

A waft of freshly-toasted bread raced up my nostrils and lanced my brain as I walked into *Bean There, Done That* just before 1 pm. Yes, my daily jaunt to the coffee store, and the first time I've noticed the smell of food. As I approach the barista girl behind the counter, the smell strengthens. Then, I register the butter and jam from someone else's order. The croissants and cakes smell lovely. In this post-lunch period, it's clear to me that *everyone but me* is enjoying their snacks and drinks.

My nostrils hadn't registered a damn thing but they're certainly processing the goodness, now. It seems the barista has remembered my request for semi-skimmed milk with my remarkably low-calorie beverage and pours it into my takeout cup. I tear the top of the sugar packet open and sprinkle about five granules into the solution, stir it around a bit, and make my way to my favorite seat outside…

… to find a girl I know as Unlucky Number 8, who I introduced you to in yesterday's entry, sitting there with her tiny Time Bandit of a buddy, and another friend of theirs I don't recognize. Unlucky Number 8 slouches in her chair and hunches her gargantuan frame over the table, presumably trying to use her overly made-up face to fight gravity. You're **Fooling Nobody** but yourself, babe, which is somewhat ironic as that's exactly the skill you need to shed a few hundred pounds. I just realized that *Babe* is rather fitting movie reference, given the circumstances…

I sit in the *opposite* chair and plug in my earphones, but Unlucky Number 8's chatter with her friend is so loud. It's the perfect opportunity to remove them and eavesdrop. They're talking about their high school days in a way that suggests they're not long out of high school. What gives that fact away? Well, they can remember each of their subject tutor's names with relative ease. I'd struggle to remember just two of my high school teacher's names at this point. Their conversation fives headfirst into an unforgiving contest between them to find the teacher they hated most.

It reminds me of a book I wrote called *Let's Kill Mr. Pond*, about two students who plot to murder their woodwork teacher. Unlucky Number 8 rattles off a list of her school's staff members and awards them a score. I swear I am not making this up or fabricating it for the sake of a narrative arc. I'll leave fate to deal with that.

One of the teachers they evaluated was "okay", according her little friend. The next teacher mentioned was described as pretty but mean. Another, allegedly, was (and presumably still is) a registered sex offender. I can't make out if "8" is kidding or not but I'm not *really* listening to what she's saying. Rather, I'm listening to *how* she's describing these teachers of hers; the speed, tone, intonation, where the lulls and dips are in her performance, so I can ascertain if she's embellishing anything. I've decided she's embellishing *a lot*. At one point her little buddy cracks a joke. She laughs, and her friend says "that's a great metaphor" only to be told by her that "no, it can't be a metaphor. It's sexual. It's a euphemism."

I find that bizarre. For a girl who's barely twenty-years-old, and pretending to find a job most days to satisfy her disappointed father, she knows that word. She's wrong, mind you. I think the term she's looking for is "innuendo" - but, credit where it's due, it's a lot better than I was expecting.

Does all this make me sound mean? Do you have any less sympathy for me for thinking - and then documenting - all this? I ask because that's exactly the question that popped into my head as her voice slowly faded to nothing as my imagination kicked in and ran riot, in tandem with my pangs of hunger.

A lack of food clearly makes you behave differently. Sure, some of it is physical. I was prepared for that. I make my living - as you probably know - from the royalties of the sales of my books. Up till now they've been 100% fiction. I depend on events such as this to create new stories. I like to think I have an active imagination. Until three years ago, I wasn't using it to its maximum capacity.

But, in the Fall of 2016, I quit teaching and chose a career that suited my strengths. Three years later, Amelia and I are (hopefully sooner rather than later) moving house.

I spent most of my adult life being a teacher. Maybe I'll tell you about my teaching days if I can find a way to tie it in with the theme at hand. Alternatively, you could get a copy of *In Their Shoes: The Teacher*, my first-ever book which details everything I went through. It's all in there.

(Sorry.)

I wasn't hungry when I arose at 11 am. I gave up listening-in to Unlucky Number 8's conversation. I downed a glass of water, had my coffee, and needed two cigarettes before I could coax my bowels into shifting. And let me tell you something. I am definitely regular with my movements, even though the quantity has been reduced. I won't go into the gory details (because quite honestly, they're not especially gory anymore) save to say I am using *much less* toilet paper.

Gone, too, is the nausea - and any notion of it. My stomach gurgled a couple of times as I sat chugging away on my cigarettes and quaffed my white Americano, but I've learned to ignore it when it happens - and it happens *not very often at all*. Maybe twice a day.

When I checked my Amazon advertising shortly before I went to the toilet, I found something interesting. Since Monday June 23rd, my sales and page reads have improved. Strange, really, because I actually haven't done much with them. Maybe the end of June signals us authors getting out of the slump? Or, perhaps - *just perhaps* - writing this journal has something to do with it.

Oh no… no… no… *you know what I'm like*. If you tell me that for every pound of body weight I lose I make *a pound* in profit then that's not good news. My God, I'll be a skeleton by the time the next Conservative leader is elected on July 22nd. You definitely do not want to get me started on politics.

I've decided that the above paragraph is nonsense. I've also decided that it's a *damn good* indication of how my thinking has changed since Monday. It's only been four days since I started this little game but it feels like six. Maybe even eight.

2 pm - lunch time.

"Welcome, Madam."

"Thank you," I say to the imaginary waiter as he brings me the menu at my computer desk. "What do you recommend today?"

"Ah, *très bien*," he quaffs with the distinction of a diplomatic, "The chef recommends the tuna in sunflower oil, a light dusting of Cayenne and black pepper, finished with four slices of a recently refrigerated Granny Smith apple, sir."

"Magic. I'll have that."

And so it was that a cold tin of tuna with a sliced apple appeared at my computer desk (sadly, where I eat, but hopefully not for much longer because we're moving house and we'll have a proper dining table) and right under my nose.

Then, it hits. It's been *eighteen hours* since I last ate! It's 2 pm now. The last thing I chewed and swallowed was a banana at 10 pm last night. In my normal "fat" life I'd never gone without eating for more than, say, five minutes. But eighteen hours?

Sometimes I impress myself. If, that is, myself is a narcissistic misanthrope hell-bent on getting rid of my "titch bits", stomach, and triple chin so he can finally see his penis without having to suck in his not-insubstantial gut.

After I wrote yesterday's entry, I went to bed hating the very thought of potatoes. I remembered the smell so distinctly that I briefly considered having tuna *twice* today in place of the potato. This happened after I wrote yesterday's entry, so I obviously couldn't include it, because it'd be weird if I finished the previous chapter with "I can't stand the smell of potato and then went to bed and fell asleep" because it would have occurred *after the fact*. I mean I'm a good writer, but not *that* good that I can bend time backwards.

I digress.

The tuna and apple lunch was absolutely fine. I've found I'm eating *even slower* than in days one, two, and three. Not only am I eating slower, but I've developed a technique with fish consummation. I do chew a little bit but I caught myself rolling the pink flesh against my upper palate with my tongue, grinding it down to nothing so I could swallow. Why was I doing that? Here's a quick hit-list as to why:

1: It was fun, like a game.

2: It felt like my entire tongue was getting some action, like some poor, malnourished fifth wheel at a food orgy getting a pity kiss.

You can't do that with an apple, though, for the record.

Another great tip I've learned is how to drink. Yeah, you're doing it wrong. Here's what you do. Take a mouthful of whatever you're drinking, and exhale all the air through your nose. Then, you swallow. Since doing that, the liquid is never in danger of going down wrong, and you don't get gas. Cool, huh? It only took me *forty fricken years* (!) to discover this. Try it next time you're drinking.

After lunch I did a huge amount of "business admin" - which is to say I attended to some of my running adverts at Amazon. It's more time-consuming, forensic, and involved than you're probably thinking. I certainly won't bore you with it so you'll just have to take my word. Also, I had to correct some errors in another book I was writing.

Now that I'm well into this journal and after today's amazing work thunderstorm, I'm finding that this *project* is making me work quicker. Good things are happening.

Here's another thing I want recorded for day four. Things are definitely getting *tighter*. Probably water-loss, but it counts. I can feel it in my face, for one thing. My clothes feel as if they're getting bigger which must be a good sign. Now, I know this is pure BS. I know it's all in my head. To anyone else it'll look like nothing has changed on the outside.

When I met my wife at the train station I was *kinda* hoping she'd look at me and say something. But she didn't.

And you know what? GOOD. I don't want her to be dishonest. It won't do either of us any favors. As I've said a few times before, I'm fueled by discouragement and nay-saying. The rebellious child in me thrives on it. When you're a teacher (or a parent), you should *never, ever* say "Hey, Timmy! Stop hitting Charlotte." Instead, try this: "Timmy? If you hit Charlotte again I'll call home and tell your mother. Your choice." Children - *and indeed adults* - react far better given a dilemma, and a consequence. More often than not they'll choose your desired course of action.

And as for the negative people in my life?

Let's say someone leaves me a one-star review for my book at Amazon. I take their name, change it slightly, and use it in a future book where the character gets tortured and killed, or something along those lines. Heaven forbid anyone who dares attack me verbally. I have a forty year arsenal of comebacks of varying degrees of lunacy and psychosis that will have you weeping for your soul, desperately hoping you'll never see me again. We're all capable of being cruel. I'll expatiate more on this in a later chapter, I'm almost certain of it.

Amelia's no exception when it comes to honesty.

We walked into the town center. She wanted to get something from a very-well-known cosmetic / pharmacy franchise store which we'll refer to as *Shoes*, for the sake of avoiding non-health-related product placement.

Now, if you're a husband - or a long-term boyfriend - you'll know as well as I do that you're going to be spending a fair amount of time waiting like a twit in a cosmetic store while your wife / girlfriend / cis-gender / attack helicopter reads every damn label on every damn blusher, or pillar of lipstick, or whatever it is. Probably for about thirty minutes or longer.

Even though you walked into the store with them, a strange thing almost always happens; the boyfriend/husband disappears, and the girlfriend/wife enters a state of heaven as she looks at all that "girlie stuff" they have now. Us men simply fade from reality like that photo of Marty McFly in *Back to the Future*... until the time comes to visit the checkout to pay for whatever she's picked up.

What I'm about to reveal next has made my week. I can't wait to share it with you.

Amelia finds what she's looking for (I think? I dunno) and we make our way to the checkout. There's a cute blond girl, maybe 5'7" in height, and certainly no older than twenty-four. We'll call her *Polly*. As Amelia drops the stuff on the counter and opens her purse, I make a generic smiley eye contact with Polly quite by accident, and she smiles right at me. The eye contact lasted about 0.0576% longer than necessary, affecting some mythical magnetism.

I look away, but not in a hurried "Sorry, love, I'm married and this is my wife" kind of way, but in a "Oh, that poster on the wall about anal wart cream looks interesting" kinda way.

As Polly deals with Amelia, it suddenly hits me - hers was no ordinary smile. I used to work in retail. A perfunctory client smile is just that - with your lips. Polly had smiled with both her lips *and* eyes. I ignored it. Thinking back on it, I suspect it was because of my confidence. Holding my head up high, chest out, the ***Fool Yourself*** method alive and well and having me believe I'd lost buckets of weight. Utter nonsense, of course, but it worked in my mind.

Suddenly, the entire world seemed brighter as we make our way to a random coffee store further up the mall. It did my ego and pride the world of good. I couldn't stop my smiling. This kind of thing never, ever, ever happened when I was gorging on double bacon cheeseburgers and prawn crackers.

The thought of potatoes and never, ever wanting to consume one ever again subsided throughout the day, thankfully, because after my shower it was dinner time. I'll talk about the food, now. With ten more days left to document, I'm in serious danger of repeating myself. Though microwaved and saggy-skinned (the potato, not me) it was perfectly fine and edible. Today I learned that I need to eat the potato before it cools down, otherwise it'll taste like an *uncooked knee* - and nobody wants that. Except maybe Hannibal Lecter.

I took a shower before dinner. The moment my clothes were off and in the laundry basket, I knew that my body had gotten tighter in places. Again, I must stress that it wasn't a massive difference, but the parts that jiggled when I moved were jiggling less. Amelia was right, in my view. Weight loss does start from the top of the body and works its way down. I can feel my jaw tightening. My usually cutesy, chubby cheeks have sunk in somewhat. It's as if the diet fairy has found the handle of a winding mechanism in my back and spun it 180 degrees, tightening my entire body. Both she (the fairy, not Amelia) and I know that the handle needs a good few revolutions - maybe a half a million or so, it feels like - before I'm at my target weight.

Showering seemed easier today, too. I could reach parts with ease that I *sort of* struggle to reach on any given kebab day. Then, I looked down the length of my body and saw something that fully confirmed my decision to never eat like fat pig again.

My pork sword.

(Or "penis", if you want the technical vernacular.)

Once again I find myself writing this entry after Amelia has gone to bed, around midnight. I'm not going to lie, I'm feeling a bit peckish right now. I had a banana at 10:30 pm. As I type this sentence it's 1:56 am on Friday. I'll hit the sack in about an hour after I've wound down and do all this again.

Four days in, and I know my appetite (and other physical things) have shrunk. I told Amelia today that I think I could do a tin of tuna and sliced apple every day now till the day I die. I'm 99% sure I could, with the exception of *maybe* one time per a month, and even then it'd be circumstantial. For example, if we're on a day trip to a theme park, or the center of London, or held captive as hostages in a siege, then I won't hunt down a tin of tuna and sliced apple. I'll just "enjoy" myself food-wise on those infrequent, but inevitable occasions.

After today, in the extremely unlikely event I feel the urge to sabotage both this project *and this book* then I'll remember Polly's smile. Thanks, Polly.

Tomorrow is Friday. It occurs to me that I've only been undertaking this project on a weekday so far. Soon it'll be the weekend. Amelia will almost surely have a Chinese takeout at some point. I'll be the one to go fetch it. Saturday is going to be unreasonably hot and humid, according to the weather report. We'll see in future entries if Amelia does have the Chinese, or an Indian, but if she thinks I'm going to snap like a fortune cookie and cave in to the taste of a chicken madras, then she's got another thing *cumin...*

Calories Consumed:

Tuna = 120

Apple = 80c

Jacket Potato = 250

Yogurt = 55

Banana = 100

3 x Coffee = 150

4 x Squash = 80

Grand Total: 840

Day 5, or:
"Five Flights"

"I'm not walking to the fifth floor.
I'd actually like to be able to speak by the time I get up there."
- Oliver Reeder, *The Thick of it* (2009)

<u>Friday, June 28th, 2019</u>

Every apple looks like mushy peas. Every potato looks like a giant French fry from the *Heart Attack Grill*. That tin of tuna? I may as well be scoffing a lump of pink, refined sugar. The yogurt I have after the potato is just animal fat - with added sugar.

That's what they look like. When they're actually in front of my eyes at the very same desk I am typing these words (where I eat), they look exactly like what they *really are*. I think it's fair to say that, now I'm five days into this journey that, not only is my body acclimatizing to this project, but *my brain is*, too.

I seldom feel hunger. It's 7:30 pm and Amelia and I are sitting outside a different branch of *Bean There, Done That* in the middle of an industrial estate that houses a few furniture showrooms and a brand new, giant supermarket we've yet to visit. I sip on my white Americano and

Amelia, tired and stressed-out from the week's work, asks me something I thought I knew the answer to - but didn't.

"Are you hungry?"

"Huh?"

"Are you hungry?"

Good question, I remember thinking. The first two days were the worst, of course. I've now got a bit of a scab where I bit into my thumb, and my little finger on the same hand now has strands of dead skin hanging from where I'd been chewing. Then, the answer finally comes to me. It went a little bit like this:

"It's kinda hard to tell," I say, with no hint of humor.

"What do you mean?"

"I've figured it out. I don't think I'm especially hungry. *I'm mistaking my salivating for being hungry.*"

There. Right there, in a nutshell. Let's explore this in a bit more detail, shall we? Think back to the last time you were hungry. Not peckish, but generally "Oh my God, I think I'm gonna die if I don't eat" kinda hungry.

The chances are that your stomach was grumbling - or at least in some state of discomfort - when you were last *truly* hungry. If your mouth is watering then you've missed the point. That's simply your brain in overdrive - making up for some fantasy of devouring whichever food you're craving.

My wife looked at me like I was some kind of idiot. I explained that I wasn't especially hungry despite the six hours that had passed since I had lunch (tuna and apple, in case you were wondering.)

We soon hit this new supermarket because Amelia wanted some groceries. She's essentially explored every single foodstuff known to man at one point or another, which is a curious counterpoint to my "I know what I like and I like what I know" attitude to food.

Among my all-time favorite foods are hamburgers, lamb kebabs, Chinese, Indian, Japanese - basically, anything that you shouldn't eat is what I love, and no exception. Dude, I'll consume it all. Each dinner in my thirties - whatever it was - was usually takeout of some description, and if not, then processed garbage. Microwavable pasta, meatballs, cheese and bacon quiches, all served with a side of fries, lovingly cooked to within an inch of their disgusting, carb-high lives.

I'll admit that that last paragraph is making my mouth water, but my brain has learned to ignore it. *Fool Yourself.* If the results of my stupid decision to undertake this decision haven't worked wonders, then at least this whole thing would have served as a testament to my BS ability.

So, as we're traversing the aisles of the supermarket, we're greeted with a special offer for eight tins of a very well-known soda. That's where it starts, you know.

I'm just like you (probably, or perhaps I should say I think you're like me?) in that I'll order a cheese and bacon half pounder with extra mayonnaise and a large fries with salt and vinegar *and* a Diet Soda. LOL. Sound familiar? Apparently, a Diet Soda is actually worse for you than regular soda because it's got all sorts of scientific nonsense in there that makes you fatter.

There's that damn word again - *diet*.

It's ridiculous, these hyper-mega-conglomerate using that word "diet" as if to mean that by drinking their product you automatically lose weight. I know, I know. From a legal standpoint they're on perfectly sound feet with that assessment. They could call it "Weight Loss Soda" and change the color from red to silver and fatties would still drink it as if it's some magic potion; that, somehow, that lone, small drink can counterbalance the impending coronary due to all those tacos you've been eating.

Unfortunately, the word "diet" has gotten such a bad rap these days that it should be banned altogether. You know I know this because I flat-out refused to refer to this two-week quest as a *diet*. Say it out loud. Spell it. Go on, I'll wait. Actually, no, hold on, I'll do it with you. Here we go…

D - I - E - T

It's the ***Fool Yourself*** thing at its height, right? Diet. What an ugly and unfeasibly unattractive proposition, right? Wantonly putting yourself through misery in order to shed a few pounds. There's no challenge in it, and little reason to see it through. It's a well-known fact in my largely unverified brain of facts that over 90% of people who lose weight put it all back on within two years.

So, here's a lasting tip I've dreamed up and plan to stick to - it's not the weight you need to lose, but your *attitude*. And I'm not just talking about your attitude to food, my friend. I'm talking about your attitude, *period*. Your attitude to food for sure but also to your physical and mental well-being, your family and friends, and your attitude to each passing hour that you're awake.

With that in mind, I stroll down the aisles for the first time since starting this project (we do our weekly food shop on a Friday) and am greeted by … oh, gosh… *absolutely everything*. Poppadums, cakes, bags of sugar, croissants, biscuits, chocolate bars, frozen boxes of all sorts of meats and culinary delights from around the world, including those I mentioned a few paragraphs above. A veritable haven of delicious food that - just last Friday - I snapped up without hesitation and dumped in our basket.

This evening, though, these aisles contain warnings. Yummy carcinogens drenched in butter - 40% off the listed price! *Bam!* Melted-cheese-pancreatic-tumor-when-you're-58-years-old-and-fries. *Wallop!* Delicious Belgian chocolate sudden stroke with your fifth bite, only $1.29.

I hung my head over the bars of the trolley as I trundled forward wondering if I'd ever eat any of the food I so dearly love. Surely I would, I thought. We reach the checkout line and I decant the items in our basket onto the conveyor belt and realize something insane.

None of these items are for me!

Pause that image of my face in shock for a second (if you need help with this, just look at the cover again - that silly cartoon is me, and it's eerily accurate.)

Huh? How can none of these items be for me?

"Andrew?"

"Yes, my darling wife?"

"Why does your face look like it's paused?"

"Because… because…"

"You said you didn't want anything?"

"I know, but…"

I told her before we entered the store (it's okay - you can hit *play* again) that I didn't need anything. We're totally stocked up on tuna and potatoes and so on. Packets of snacks and various other items shuffling along towards the cute checkout girl are *all* for Amelia, and not one thing is for me.

Nothing for me? Pfft. Being married, I'm well-versed with that particular experience, and I have fully accepted it.

On the drive home I remember to tell Amelia something I'd done during the day.

"What?" she asked.

"I used the stairs instead of the elevator, today."

"Oh."

Rewind... back to 1:45 pm this afternoon when I drove back from my daily dalliance at *Bean There, Done That*. Yes, Unlucky Number 8 was there, before you ask and - yes - she was with her tiddly sidecar of a friend talking some nonsense about something or other. I dunno, I gave up listening. It was an incredibly lovely day today. The wind had died down. The sun was shining and there were only *two* - count 'em, *two* - tables in the shade under the canopy. Somehow, that over-sized behemoth and her five chins managed to take up the *entire* table and an extra seat for her fat, tree trunk of a leg.

I really like Unlucky Number 8, in case you hadn't noticed. She brightens up my day. I suppose it goes some way to prove that a fat girl who's as ugly on the inside as she is on the outside faces that age-old, unsolvable jigsaw; she may one day be thin, but she'll always be a nasty and prejudicial loser. Potatoes and tuna may change her frame but won't improve her character or attitude.

Or will it?

After all, it seems to be changing my character to a degree. I'll go into that later because I don't want to speak too soon - and the jury is still out on that. Look, if we get to chapter ten and I've not brought it up, can you remind me? Thanks.

So, *stairs*. Big deal, I hear you think with your cranium. But not if you live on the fifth floor of an apartment block. I didn't count each set of stairs, but there must be ten per flight or something close. I'll make sure to check tomorrow when I do it again.

The fifth floor of our apartment block is *really, really* quite high. If I were to fall off my balcony - and believe me, I nearly have a few times - I wouldn't survive the impact on the road one hundred feet below. It's not a case of my breaking my legs, more a case of an overweight mass of cheeseburgers and biscuits exploding like a blood-stuffed cantaloupe. So, you know, it's rather high up.

I climbed the first and second sets of stairs and find myself on the third floor fairly arrogant and full of myself. "Meh, that was cool."

The fourth floor… and my legs are starting to throb like a thumb after a car door has been slammed shut on it. I dread the thought of going up the last flight to the fifth and final floor, but I manage it and need to pause for a break to catch my breath. It's not *as bad* as it surely reads, but a little five-second break was required.

Fortunately, the door to our apartment is right next to the case so no one sees just how out of breath / shape / my mind I truly am. You know when you sort of suck your breath in and act all cool when you're out of breath? Yeah, *that*.

My legs continued to throb for about two minutes. I found that part of my brain that concentrates all the exhaustion and out-of-breath-near-heart-attack-ness to my thighs and away from my chest and face. **Fool Yourself** achievement unlocked: Grand Master! It's true. You can concentrate pain and exhaustion to certain areas of your body if you're really, really in tune with your own mind. There must be something in it, surely?

As a former teacher I can promise you that everything is an act. I spent six months being nervous before walking into a classroom until, one day, I just thought "ah, whatever," and *acted* confident. Oh, there's that I planned to do that until I became confident. But you know something funny? The act became me. I never grew confident. It was just a *version* of me my students were getting; a confident, fictional character called Andrew Mackay - one who took very little nonsense and had a totally different approach to teaching. A fine example of **Fool Yourself** working a little *too* well.

The same thing is happening here with this dangerously low-calorie intake I've entertained for the fifth day running.

After I finished lunch (go on, have a guess what it was. Oh, I already told you a few paragraphs ago, sorry) my right hand, quite without my permission, clicked on the mouse and took me to a leading online retailer beginning with the letter "A". I'll give you a clue - it's very likely where you got this book from.

I then found myself typing "exercise gear" and was somewhat surprised to find that I was looking at thigh masters and such. It's weird when you're an author who sells their books on Amazon (did you get the answer correct? Yay!) and become the customer. You look at the site differently. Dear reader, you've probably no idea what I'm talking about, but when I go to Amazon it's usually to check my reviews, or to risk re-reading my product description and praying there are no embarrassing literacy errors.

You, on the other hand, don't know that feeling (unless you're a fellow author buddy reading this, in which case 'hello') and are used to being a customer. I fastidiously - and with severe prejudice - check out the reviews on all these items. Also worth looking at is the rank. Just how popular is the item doing in comparison with others of its type? I want quality, inexpensiveness, and a Prime Delivery option so I can have Mr. Bezos himself operate his trillion-dollar time machine no-one knows about and get what I just ordered to me *yesterday*.

I find what I'm looking for. Something called a Power Bar. A big stick thing with a coiled middle that sort of bends into a C shape. You use it with your arms. It's meant to tone and shape your arms and chest. Good, because I'm fed up with having breasts like Dolly Parton's in her prime.

Oh, I also order two hand grips, too, because, you know, I'm a writer with an evident comma complex, if this particular sentence, is anything, to go, by. I figure those squeezy hand things that help your wrist muscle up might come in handy for writing on my keyboard, and not another activity associated with wrists, *thank-you-very-much*. If you're appalled by that PG-rated innuendo (which, as we learned the other day is what it is, courtesy of Unlucky Number 8) then *I seriously advise you not to buy* a book called "The Chrome Junction Academy Trilogy" by yours truly. It's ridiculously offensive and funny. You can get it at Amazon… *while I stop typing and go for a smoke*.

Ah, that's better.

Oh. I just remembered something important while I was smoking on the balcony. I hired this really cool artist called Gary to do the illustration for this book cover. I drew a sketch of what I wanted and sent it to him with some style examples. We should hopefully see the first iteration of it on Sunday. Ooo, exciting!

Wow, this chapter is already 2,522 words and I only started typing 45 minutes ago. I think I'm rambling. I don't get to speak to too many people with my mouth in my line of work, but I am a rambler. I'm sure by now you've noticed I don't (and have never) suffered from writer's block. My mind is wandering. It's almost 1 am and I'm just typing. My brain has taken leave of my body and I am literally just watching my fingers dance on the keyboard. There it is again. *And again.*

Okay, a couple of quick things to note before I finish writing this entry and go and amuse myself before bed.

France broke a weather record today. It hit 46 Celsius (114.8 F) - their hottest day since records began. People died - something to do with an African plume of bottled gas traveling over the Mediterranean. Tomorrow is set to the hottest day of the year for us in the UK. Our heat is stifling and humid, unlike, say, California's dry heat. They're advising us to close the windows and huddle in the bathroom till it's over.

Not me, though. I have an appointment with *Bean There, Done That* at lunchtime. The tuna isn't refrigerated in our apartment.

And additional point to note is that tomorrow is *not* a weekday. It's Saturday, so Amelia is home. Presumably on the sofa with the fan on and keeping as cool (and endowed, for fear of missing a blatantly crass innuendo) as a cucumber.

A part of me is hoping I wake up like *Slenderman* so I can roll up to the shopping mall topless and have all the ladies make eyes at me.

The other part of me hopes that the project can survive my wife being at home cooking all sorts of stuff.

I'll see you tomorrow.

Calories Consumed:

Tuna = 120

Apple = 80c

Jacket Potato = 250

Yogurt = 55

Banana = 100

3 x Coffee = 150

3 x Squash = 60

Grand Total: 820

Day 6, or:
"A Fung Guy to be With"

"Start the process of self-control with some penance; begin with fasting."
- Mahavira

<u>Saturday, June 29th, 2019</u>

What are the health implications of consuming less than one thousand calories per day? I mean I feel fine, but what if something happens further down the road? What can I do about it? Nothing.

At least when they find my corpse they'll only need two men to lift me up, and not four.

I ask the first question because today, the hottest day of the year so far (34C / 93.2), Amelia said my face had turned all yellow - with a pink outer edge. I put the pink down to having caught the sun. I'm naturally fair in both complexion and hair, so I burn like a round wicker basket the moment I'm out of the shade. It was blindingly hot today and my regular trip to *Bean There, Done That* allowed me a few seconds in the sun. Jeez, the sun was a scorcher. I remember last year I visited Los Angeles and Las Vegas.

The sun in Las Vegas will kill most Brits if they stay in it long enough. We're used to rain and clouds, you see.

But my face? I confess, when I looked in the mirror I couldn't really see any 'yellow'. Perhaps it was the lighting in the room? Who knows. I told her I felt fine (and not especially hungry, as it happens) and we kind of left it at that. But it did make me think.

I took lunch a bit later than usual today. I don't know why. I woke up just before 11 am and did my morning ritual, as always. Amelia was on the sofa and enjoying the fan blowing cool air on her. I suggested we shut the windows and close the blinds to contain the cool air. It worked a treat.

I ended up watching an hour-long YouTube video with magician Penn Jillette being interviewed by a woman. Fascinating stuff. This led to me watching a TED Talk on dieting, and another, until such time as two hours flew by with my YT-hopping. Eventually, I happened upon a video about Intermittent Fasting (IF) and ketosis. A highlight was a video called Therapeutic Fasting by someone named Dr. Jason Fung. I'll include it in the links and references at the end of this book.

After I returned from *Bean There, Done That* (yeah, Unlucky Number 8 was there as usual and hogging the one good seat in the shade, since you ask) I had my usual drink. For the first time, on day six, I wasn't even hungry for it. It might have been due to the weather. I wasn't hungry at all. I'm not in the business of starving myself to death. I figured I needed the protein if nothing else, and so ate my tuna lunch very slowly whilst watching a TED Talk on

"The Second Brain"; an essay on how microbes and bacteria actually inform our thinking. It took forty minutes to eat lunch, which I did very, very slowly.

All the videos I'd seen about dieting and so on led me to have a bizarre idea. This *fasting* thing Dr. Jason Fung talks about. He's saying we're doing it all wrong - that "eat less, move more" is a myth and doesn't work. He's provided a lot of compelling evidence. What if I eat *nothing*, say, this coming Monday? July 1st. The halfway point of this project? There was a video about the benefits of fasting (admittedly aimed at women) but, since I have impressive breasts anyway, I figure it could be worth a shot? Right?

It's Sunday tomorrow. No doubt I'll have made up my mind about any commitment to fasting by then. I'm 50 / 50 on it to be perfectly honest with you. Then, there was a news story today about a man whose wife is holed up in a jail cell in Iran, or somewhere like that. He sat outside the Iranian embassy in London and went on hunger strike along with his wife in order to draw attention to their cause. I forget their names, but this is a pretty big story right now in the UK. They were on hunger strike for *fifteen days*!! It seems they drank water (and in his case, a large espresso, judging by the news media footage) but did not eat.

Well, well, well… if they can go fifteen days without solids, then surely I can? Right?

Ah, you know what? Screw it. I've decided I'll do it. That news story coupled with the science behind fasting has sold me.

In two days' time, on Monday July 1st, I will only consume filtered water (and certainly forgo the Cordial/squash) and black coffee without the three granules of sugar. A complete and utter detox right at the halfway mark of this two-week journey. Wonderfully enough I can *still* go to *Bean There, Done That*. I'll just have black coffee and no creamer. Be gone, toxins!

The odds of my dying from fasting appear to be pretty slim (ho-ho!) and, to you, the fact that you're reading this journal suggests that I survived it, right? Ha. Not necessarily so. How would you feel if you got to next Wednesday to find a message from my author friend who's going to give you bad news and published this book on my behalf?

I have something pretty interesting to report to you, too. When I got back from *Bean There, Done That*, I took the stairs to our apartment on the 5th floor like I did yesterday. This time, I counted how many steps it took. Each flight has eighteen concrete steps.

So, here's a little mathematical equation.

Five floors, obviously, but from the ground to the 1st floor is actually 24 steps.

18 x 5 + 24 = 114 steps

It gets better, though. I actually achieved this feat *three times* today. Once, after I got back from the coffee store, once after I went downstairs to run a few errands, and *a third time*, after I went to the movie theater. I climbed 342 steps today. Large, unforgiving concrete steps, and I didn't use the handrail, either.

The first time I did it my legs weakened around the second level. I had to take a break at the third level. The last time I did it I managed to go from the car park (sorry, didn't count the steps, but there aren't that many) and managed to sprint up to the fourth floor and take a few seconds to catch my breath, and then continue at a bit of a slower pace.

Amelia wanted to know why I was out of breath when I walked through the door. So, I told her. I also revealed something I decided about 0.098 seconds before I said it, which was that - from this moment on - I will always take the stairs unless we have heavy groceries or we return to the apartment block together. I figure I'll be doing the climb at least twice per day, now.

Let's rewind to earlier this morning (barely, it was about 11:50 am) when I had consumed half of my morning coffee and sucked in the first cigarette of the day.

I sat on the toilet seat ready to rock and roll and noticed something *really* peculiar. The toilet seat appeared to have widened - not just a little bit but *a lot bit*, by all accounts. Where the plastic usually rides up a certain area of my buttocks (you know what I'm talking about and don't deny it!) the sides have now slid up around the curvature. Not by inches, of course, but noticeable enough for it register. Taking a dump never felt so confirmatory, or great, I must admit. I was *sure* that things were getting tighter. My wobbly bits wobbling less, and so on. My face has definitely tightened despite Amelia's insistence that she can't see it. She can see it in the same way we never notice our spouses or kids aging subtly over the years. She's the most subjective person in this process and, it must be said, the *only* one who knows I'm doing it - and the only reason she knows is because I'm more likely to get away with an affair (chances of that = 0%, by the way) than her noticing I've changed my ~~diet~~ approach to nutrition.

Ugh. I just re-read those last few words. *Now I'm starting to sound like them.* You know, those annoying dietitians. Look at me; like some kind of pap scientist bettering himself like a complete and utter bore. Yawn.

I'm sorry if these entries / this book reads like the ramblings of a madman. Actually, I'm not sorry. It's frank and in-the-moment. My mind tends to wander and get all creative and stuff. If you're looking for your next read, then if you check out my fiction, you'll see it's all carefully constructed and perfectly formed. This work, however, is more scatter-brained than that. If I black out from a lack of fish next Thursday I'll still type my entry but there's a serious risk that it might come out as double dutch wrapped in gobbledygook. For that I make no apology.

See, I learned something important today. It kind of goes some way to answering that question absolutely nobody keeps asking me: "Do you think your weight loss changes your attitude and thinking." Well, here's something I think I believe in now. Ready, here goes…

Don't eat for fun.

Simple, right? Everything we put in our bodies should, first and foremost, be at the service of nutrition - and nutrition alone. Are you eating that cheeseburger because you're hungry, or you just like the taste? In your mind you've already said "both" (I'm psychic like that) but which is the priority?

Okay, I'm getting ahead of myself. Let me explain. This whole ordeal is going to finish at midnight on Sunday, July 7th. That *doesn't* mean at 00:01 on Monday, July 8th I am going to gorge on "Diet Soda", Pringles, and Chunky Kit Kats - and I promise you, our cupboard is *still* chock-full of those very items. I know they're there, and I like that. It means every time I am tempted to pop till I can't stop, I won't. You know how many times since Monday I've thought about going into the cupboard to get one of those items?

None.

So, I'm now thinking long-term. The first three days were a psychological exercise for me - to reduce my appetite. I think it's worked well. That 72-hour period might have planted a tumor in my pancreas that'll make itself known, erupt, and advance to stage 4 around November of the year 2038. Maybe it won't. Who the hell knows? It'll have twenty-year build-up of tar and nicotine to contend with, anyhow.

I think I've mentioned this before but, in case I haven't, I'll say it again - on Monday night of July 8th, I plan to have a lamb kebab and chips, drenched in garlic mayo and chili sauce with little in the way of lettuce and cabbage. And a soda of some description. It'll be the last entry in the diary. I won't have lunch that day, either, just for fun. I need to weigh myself that morning, too, so please remind me.

Back to the matter at hand, though… what's the long-term solution to continue my weight-loss? After Monday? I'm sure it'll involve beans, vegetables, whole plants, and maybe some brown rice. Jacket potatoes and tuna like sounds a good bet. I've been tempted to mix them, but I won't. Not just yet, anyway.

Maybe a light quiche? I think a modest curry might go down well. Even the odd chicken wrap or fish supper. I'm not a vegan, and I doubt I'll ever be one because I like meat too much. And bacon, obviously. Okay, so here's what I'm thinking, just bear with me…

As of the morning of Tuesday July 9th, I will only consume around 2,000 calories per day *for the rest of my natural life*. "What?!" I hear you say. "Ah," I respond in kind, "You haven't heard the good bit, yet…"

Calories are calories, whichever way you slice and pan-fry them. So one calorie in a chicken kebab is the same as one calorie in a strawberry. It's the nutrition that counts. "Good fat" vs "bad fat", for example.

So, we all know by now that before dinner - if I keep up the tuna thing, or some variant of it (e.g. tuna and a banana instead of apple etc) - then by dinnertime, I'll have only consumed about 300 calories when you factor in the coffee and Cordial/squash addition to my water.

I know some days I can miss lunch. We'll prove that on *both* Monday - the first *fast* Monday, and the second

Monday, which we'll call *Andrew is a disgusting, fat-quitter "Kebab Monday"*.

That means I have roughly 1000 calories to spend on whatever I damn well please for dinner, to ensure I fall within the 1500+ calorie bracket.

Now, I'm not suggesting I'm going to eat burgers and chips every night because that's just stupid. More often than not I'll plump for something healthy and certainly not processed. More on that later, because I need time (probably next week) to draw up a list of stuff I can have. Variety is key to this whole endeavor working. Wanna know why? Because I'm a realist, and I know myself better than anyone else. Seriously, I know stuff about me you guys don't. It would shock you to know some of those things, so don't ask. We've all asked our friends and family that age-old question: "if you could only eat one food for the rest of your life what would it be?" We tend to respond with imaginative answers like "Chicken," or "Hamburgers," or "Daisy Ridley," or… hang on, I think I might have to revisit that last one. If you tell me I can only eat a potato for the rest of my life I'd have never started this stupid gig in the first place. Similarly, if you told me I could *never, ever* eat a kebab ever again in my life, I'd just decide to stay obese. There's no question of it.

Fortunately, this isn't what I am proposing. What I *am* proposing is this:

I *think* Monday might be my fasting day. One day to let my system chew away at the stored fat for the previous week. Coffee and water only. Detox. But, and here's the clincher, I can have *one* takeout each week as well. It's likely to be a Saturday for a couple of reasons:

1: Wife is home, and loves takeout, and,

2: The Chinese takeout place is closed on a Sunday.

Does this trade-off sound wise? One day of fasting so I can have one evening of bad food? In theory it sounds great. Sure, in theory, I'm 160 lbs in the not-too-distant future, and have a line of super models begging to bury their head between my brilliantly svelte thighs. *In theory.*

In practice? Nothing worth doing was ever easy, remember that. I need to road test *fasting*; this even-sillier-idea-than-the-original-idea out, first, to see if I can stand it, which is why Monday July 1st is my trial run.

This reads more like a tantrum than an entry for today's shenanigans. I've covered the main parts already, but I would like to leave you with this final thought.

What if I told you that this is all achievable and you *could* actually eat whatever / whenever you want and still lose weight? Yeah, I know, if you watch Jillette's Big think YouTube video, he says the same thing, but he goes onto say that what he *wants* has changed significantly. He can eat as many Brussels Sprouts and lettuce leaves as he wants, sure.

I'll drop this thought in your head. I need to ask you a question. What's your favorite *bad* food? Chocolate cake? Something cheese-based? Pick one that's notorious for clogging arteries. It's okay, I'll wait.

Okay, got one in mind?

I'll go with chocolate cake because I (think I still) really like it. Here's where we come full circle and ask the question:

Why are you eating it?

I'm guessing it's not for the nutrition. Rather, it's for the taste. It can't be for the impending rumble of diabetes or the fluffy addition to your muffin top, right? Nah, it's definitely for the taste.

The last time you ate <insert your choice here> how much of it did you have? I dunno about you, but if chocolate cake is anything like cigarettes, the *first* puff / bite / swallow / inhale of the day is the best, and subsequent bites/puffs just don't live up to that initial intake. A bit like when you have sex with someone for the first time. Sure, the second, third, fifteenth, twenty-fifth encounter is great. But what about the six-thousand-two-hundred-and-twenty-seventh time? Not that I've been counting. Actually, thinking about it, there'd be nothing left of Amelia - or my anatomy - if we'd clock that kind of mileage, but the point still stands.

Here's what you do. Buy the <insert answer here> anyway. And, if it's the chocolate cake, here's what you do. Cut just enough of the cake - maybe the size of a credit card - and treat your taste buds. Put the rest away.

Sounds like a good idea. It's a *dangerous* idea. Once you pop etc. It'll work amazingly well for some. It'll feel as if you're never on a diet. At least your tongue and belly will think you're not dieting - and that's half the battle won, right there. The art of *Fool Yourself*: **Taste Bud Edition.** For others, it'll be the death of them - maybe literally. The adventure to slim down and eat healthy will be over.

I like to think I know which of those two categories I fall into.

I'm not sure if I even need to try, though.

Calories Consumed:

Tuna = 120

Apple = 80c

Jacket Potato = 250

Yogurt = 55

Banana = 100

3 x Coffee = 150

3 x Squash = 60

Grand Total: 820

Day 7, or:
"The Lazy Route"

"Jason, I mean there's something alive in Yogurt. It's called benign
bacteria. I mean, under a microscope you can see them moving, so
what's the difference? They're good for us, Jason.
They kill the bad things inside us."
- Jason's Father, *The Stuff* (1985)

<u>*Sunday, June 30th, 2019*</u>

I woke up nervous today about the decision I told you
about yesterday - *fasting*. I couldn't stop thinking about it.
Truly, food for thought (and not belly, for once!) and I
wasn't even hungry when I woke up at 11 am. It was much
cooler than Saturday, which, as I may have mentioned, was
the hottest day of the year for the UK. A thought occurred
to me this afternoon when I was having my daily coffee at
Bean There, Done That - I'm kinda glad I decided to do this
project during the hottest period of the year. What if I'd
done it in Winter? With the Christmas break and all the
turkey and trimmings? It'd have been a disaster, I think.

For all intents and purposes, I'm halfway through this
whole ordeal. Actually, calling it an ordeal is completely off
the mark. It's been remarkably easy, actually. I've decided

that the third and fourth day were the worst and, thinking back to Wednesday and Thursday, they were pretty awful.

I *am* going to fast tomorrow. I want to prove I can do it. It's not some feeble-minded attempt to say that humans don't require food, or that it's a waste of money, but I am very curious to learn about myself. Can I do it? I think I have a fighting chance. Also, I need to record *why* I'm doing it in the first place, so I figure here is as good a place as any.

Before I go into the whys and wherefores of this decision, I'll tell you how today went down - because honestly there's not very much to report. I noticed for the first time today that getting up from my work chair is a lot easier now. I think about it less. I fear less for my back with ordinary, everyday movements. Also - and this is the golden egg - when I got into my car *after* my trip to *Bean There, Done That*, I noticed that my belly wasn't protruding as much as it did a week ago. I felt the sides of the upholstery in the seat *surround* my ass rather than prop it up. Securing my safety belt was a lot easier, too. As a matter of fact, general movement is easier, now.

One of the main questions I *don't* get asked (because nobody knows I'm doing this thing) is "are you smoking more cigarettes now to compensate for the food reduction?" To my amazement, the answer is *no*. I'm still on roughly twenty coffin nails per day. Amazing, isn't it? I can count how many steps there are between my car and my apartment on the 5th floor but I don't count my cigarettes. Ah, I dunno. Who cares? I've no cause to argue with that fact. Hand, mouth, lips, suck… well, it's sort of like eating. Purely psychological no doubt - as will be the time when I eventually quit.

Another thing that punched me in the face and demanded my attention were the commercial breaks as I listened to the radio. Right now McDonald's really have mastered the desire to tempt us into their stores with something called the Chicken Flamin' Wrap-of-the-Day, or whatever it's called. I used to eat them as a snack, along with a double cheeseburger at around midnight on maybe one night in ten. And I drove to the drive thru, too, when I might otherwise have walked. I can't believe I did that. No wonder I piled on the pounds. Of course, McDonald's isn't the *only* commercial. There are Indian restaurant commercials and buy-one-get-one-frees on mayonnaise at a lower-end supermarkets.

Ordinarily, I'd be tempted. Now, I treat these commercials the same way I treat most everything in my life - including my previous profession; as *satire*. After forty years converting oxygen into carbon dioxide, you tend to take a view on things. If I've learned *one* thing (and I haven't) since the day I escaped from my mother's birth canal it's this: *Nobody knows what they're doing.*

Like, *at all.* Everyone is winging it. Yes, even *you* - and you know it, and you know that I know you know it, too.

Think about your first day at your job. Did you know what you were doing? Nope. Well, *not really.* You had to learn the rules and get shown how stuff works. Did you improve at your job? Sure you did. That's right, you did something *wrong* and either got told off by your boss or, perhaps more effectively, you kept quiet, and hoped your manager wouldn't find out. After that near-miss, you vowed never to make the same mistake again.

Now, here you are four days / weeks / months / years / decades later, still *unfired* because you're a damn good apologist or excellent at concealing all those mistakes you made. What else is there about your job or career that you don't know? Ah, that age-old adage of "I don't even know what I don't know" rears its head now only to get punched by me and sent packing. What you *don't* yet know about your job you'll soon discover when you make the mistake of handling it incorrectly. If you get to handle it again, *handle it better*; avoid making the same mistakes and expect a different outcome? You dummy. Look, we're all going to be just *fine*. But I'm afraid neither of us still knows what we're doing.

Agreed? Good, we can move on with our lives.

Before lunch I had something of a very light dizzy spell. The balcony began to spin and my thighs seemed to weaken. Do you want to know how I made it stop? I shut my eyes and groaned and finally said "Oh, grow up," albeit with a couple more R-rated curse words.

It stopped almost immediately. Amazing. That's some dense psychology for someone way more qualified than me to analyze. Telling my ills to go away? What nonsense. But, you know, **Fool Yourself**, and everything. See, what works for me might not work for you, so don't get your hopes up, my friend.

Now to the interesting parts of the day.

My wife and I went to the local shopping mall (which isn't very far from our apartment block) so she could buy some stuff from *Shoes*. We did that, and then went for a coffee. I had my usual, and she had… *whatever*. On the way back we stopped by a local convenience store and filled up a plastic bag with snacks and stuff for her dinner.

Then (drum roll) I had an idea. Amelia asked me if I wanted to take the elevator. That was the *last* thing I wanted to do. See, earlier, I bought a 2.5 kg sack of potatoes for you-know-what (and if you don't *know-what* then you've clearly not been paying attention so far) and drove back home. I carried that heavy sack o' spuds up to the fifth floor in my left arm with my door key in my right hand. I was still out of breath as I reached my floor but, somehow, the steps seemed familiar. Like an old, concrete friend, whose primary concern is for me to lose weight. I can't actually foresee a time when I won't be using those stairs. Actually I can. It'll be the day we *finally* bloody move to our new house. Or unless I am zapped of energy. Our new house has a few stairs, though, so we're all good.

I've decided to call using the stairs instead of the elevator *The Lazy Route*. When I enter into the building, I look at the elevator, shoot right past it, and say "Nah, I'm taking *The Lazy Route*, mate." I know, I know. It's gotten to the point where I'm talking to inanimate machinery. That's usually the first sign of madness. Maybe I should use that for the book's product description, somewhere?

So, the second time I took *The Lazy Route* - this time, I tell my wife "Yes, I'd like to take the stairs." She grabbed the bag and said "okay" and I insisted I take the bag with me because I'd already done it with the potatoes earlier in the day. Sunday was becoming something of a "not only are you taking *The Lazy Route* but you're also carrying heavy items" day.

Because I'd set myself this task it automatically became a challenge. What if… what if… *I ascended the stairs so fast that I actually beat Amelia in the elevator?*

WOW! That's all I needed. What a great story for *The Hunger Diaries*, too! So, I raced up the stairs with the heavy bagful of noodles and chocolate (I dunno what was in it) and ran as fast as I could whilst Amelia took the elevator. I made it to the fourth floor before I had to catch my breath, but even then it was only for three seconds. I mentally pushed through the pain in my thighs and raced up the next flight. All the while, the concrete wall turned transparent, revealing an image of Amelia trapped in a metal cage flying up faster than I could run. There was simply no way in hell she was gonna beat me to our apartment.

I push several pain barriers and made it to the fifth floor. In my own silly mind of course, I knew I hadn't beaten the elevator. I mean I'm good… but I'm not *that* good. Wouldn't it be lovely, though, if I burst through the door to our apartment and met Amelia as she was trundling down the corridor to our front door? Answer: yes, it would.

It didn't happen, though.

Out of breath, I walked into our apartment to find Amelia already doing other stuff. It seemed she'd been there a while. She popped her head out of the bedroom door and said, simply, "Hmm. Not bad."

Not bad?

That was flippin' EPIC, by the way. What do you mean it was "not bad"? I thought as I smiled and acted as if I wasn't peeved off.

I lost the race by at least two minutes, probably more. Please, don't tell me one day I'll win it else I'll have to train for it. Besides, I had a disadvantage, didn't I? I was carrying something heavy. "Yeah, *my own flabby gut and breasts*," the little voice inside your head when you read a book screams.

Believe me, I'm receiving that snarky voice loud and clear.

Shower time. I don't shower every single day but I'm not exactly a Neanderthal, either. Once every two or three days. Why? I'm lazy, honestly. But I like to think it's to preserve my own bodily smells and man musk to make me more attractive to the female species. You can take that answer however you like, but I can't guarantee the taste shouldn't be at least a little salty.

Last week I didn't particularly love to shower. It's a pain in the buttocks, really, isn't it? And it's boring. Well, not while you're going through *The Hunger Diaries*. My legs and ass are definitely… *squeezed*. Oh, don't get me wrong, I'm not going to be appearing on the cover of *Vogue* anytime soon, but they're definitely getting there. Time to lose a bit of groin fat, too, or the *pushin' cushin'* as my wife has never referred to it as because she doesn't have a warped sense of humor or filthy mind like I do.

I'm looking forward to showering now for reasons that must be patently obvious to you as a reader. It affords me the chance to really explore my body in extremely unforgiving conditions. The harsh fluorescent lighting, the giant mirror above the sink, and I'm all slippery and wet and stuff. I know my body very well (some parts more than others) and each time I *have* to touch it I can feel a difference. Oh, also - get this - the towel is covering *more* of my thighs, too. The two ends meet quite comfortably. I've used less of the towel to dry myself. Just *one* week into the stupid adventure and I'm seeing results. Would you like a bonus result, too? Get this… my spectacles are starting to slide off my head a little bit. Especially when I look down over my balcony. Evidently, my *head* is starting to shrink.

Dinner rolls round at 8 pm. The menu, whilst decently presented, was limited to two things. Oh, go on then, I'll have the chef's special. Potato and light yogurt. I eat dinner quicker than I eat lunch and finish around 8:30 pm.

As I type this very sentence at 1:14 am on Sunday, July 14th, it hits me that I have not eaten for five hours. So far I've had a banana as a light "snack" around 10 or 11 pm so I don't go to bed hungry. I skipped the banana tonight in mini-preparation for tomorrow, which is an excellent segway into what I'd like to talk to you about.

Fasting.

Now, I'm no nutritionist as you know. For the record, I have a PGCE (Post-Grad Certificate in Teaching, which is the equivalent of a Master's Degree) and a Bachelor of Arts in Media and Film Production. So, if there's anyone qualified to talk about science and metabolism and stuff then it's certainly not me. I failed science quite spectacularly at high school and have maintained a healthy ignorance of it ever since, despite writing a best-selling, sci-fi fantasy series set in space called *Star Cat* which you should buy and read right now. Actually, I'll put a glorious and shameless advert for it right at the end of the book.

I watched a Joe Rogan YouTube video on fasting. To be honest, fasting was always kind of on my radar whenever I thought about dieting over the years. If you total up all the minutes I've spent thinking about improving my physicality and health you'll find I've spent more time vomiting. It's just that simple. As you know, my goal is to get *not fat* anymore. My target weight is twelve stone, dead. I want a BMI of no more than 24 - whatever the hell that number actually means. My goal was to reduce my appetite first, shrink my stomach (the psychological equivalent of having a stomach sleeve fitted) so I would eat less. I can say right now without fear of ~~contraception~~ contradiction that, not only has my appetite shrunk to that of an eight-year-old's, but also my taste buds have been all but reset. At least, I *think* this is the case. It sure feels like it, and I think that's all that counts. Even though I've just said it could all be BS I still believe it. Oh, hello **Fool Yourself.** How's it, uh... *hanging*? Funny how the mind works, really.

So, appetite shrunk. I get full faster. Consuming low calorie and low carbohydrates, offset with milk in my coffee and a small broadcast of sugar. Where now?

Well, I need to burn fat.

I'll pause here and take you to a brief exchange I had whilst drinking coffee with Amelia an hour before dinner.

"So, I had an idea."

"Andrew, can you *please* not start your sentence with 'so'? It's irritating. You're better than that."

"I'm sorry."

"That's okay," Amelia said. "Just don't do it again."

"Understood."

"Good. What were you saying?"

"So, I decided I want to hit my target weight of 12 stone before my 41st birthday."

"Oh. Okay. When is that?"

"Huh?" I blurted with a hint of disbelief, "It's in October, same as always. FFS."

Amelia shrugs as if to say, "Whatever, good luck."

It's technically July 1st as I'm writing which means I have three months and six days to hit twelve stone (167 lbs, 76 kg). Can I do it? Who the hell knows but it'll be fun to try.

So, as I say (I'll stop starting sentences with 'so' now, because people who do that should be dragged into the nearest parking lot and shot in the back of the head) I need to burn fat, and not burn water. See, I've learned today that this distinction is very important and the number one (or was it twelfth?) reason *blubbernaughts* fail to lose their "titch bits" (and other, embarrassing wobbly body parts) only try in earnest for a few days, and then succumb to the cake and pies.. They see some initial results; they feel a shrink and think it's working. Two days later when they climb onto the scales… three days later… a month later, perhaps… nothing. No weight lost.

Game over, fatty.

Not me, though. I'm going to be burning *fat*. It's the single-most effective way to… well, uh, lose fat. Kinda the whole point of this thing.

I learned the method I'm about to undertake off of the interwebs, so it *must* be true. Actually, my teacher instincts kicked in, and I went to a few sources to corroborate what I'd learned, as per my vow #2 in the introduction.

It turns out that if you don't eat for sixteen hours (water aside) your body burns fat and not the stuff it extracted from the food you ate. In other words, if there is no food left to burn, it'll burn the fat storage in different parts of your body. Or something like that.

Anyway, the takeaway from this is down to something called TRE, or Time-Restricted Eating. Apparently the 16:8 method is the best start. 16 hours fast, 8 hours feed.

What this means is that you have an eight-hour window to consume whatever you're eating (obviously not hot chocolate fudge or a KFC Double Artery Stack Clogger with gravy and biscuits) and then, for sixteen hours, you are not to eat anything at all. And the great thing about the sixteen-hour window is that you're probably going to sleep during it. So, it sounds more palatable, for want of a better word.

Now, here's a revelation for you. It turns out that, quite by accident, I already *have* been fasting every day since Monday! If you look at your own schedule you may find you're already doing it, too. Amazing, isn't it? A pure fluke. I get up at 11 am, and have my first coffee (it counts because of the milk and tiny bit of sugar) around 11:30 am and then have dinner around 7:30 or 8 pm. So, that's the eight hour window. I've slightly ruined it by having a banana at 10 pm (ish) but I didn't have one today.

I figure an eight-hour window is perfectly doable every day for me, essentially because I'm fortunate enough not to have to commute to work. Don't get me wrong. I work hard at my business (more than I ever did as a teacher) because I give a damn about my success as an author. I don't consider it work, though, because I'm doing something I love. The point is that I am fortunate enough to be in the position I am to enable me to undertake this ~~diet~~ project. I heard shift workers and nurses are the worst affected by their feeding schedules. Their diets and mealtimes in general are all messed up, and - as a result - they're more prone to heart attacks, strokes, and scores of other wonderful ways to shuffle off this mortal coil.

When I was a teacher, I would very infrequently eat once a day because I was so damn busy. Get up, have a coffee - or sixteen - but never eat. Dinner time would usually be a takeout after the forty-five minute walk back to my old apartment. So, because of the nutritional abstinence and power-walking I was in a severe calorie deficit before the waft of the half pounder ever hit my nostrils at the fast food joint.

Thanks, teaching, for keeping me thin - and very nearly killing me (!)

The point is I *know* I can fast. Tomorrow is my first stab at a 24 hour fast. I'm expecting pangs of hunger around 2 pm and maybe 8 pm, but they will subside. I'll down a glass of filtered water to satiate myself and reduce the hunger. You know like when you're *soooo* tired that you actually become more alert? Yeah, like that, but with hunger.

I'm going to storm right through. Also, I'm going to *walk* the two miles to *Bean There, Done That* tomorrow (unless it rains) so I can get some exercise in. Why not? We're experiencing glorious weather right now. It'll be nothing too strenuous; the walk is mostly flat except for a bit of a hill right at the end.

During a fast you're allowed a black coffee (no creamer or sugar) and water. As much of those as you like. That suits me. I still get to go to the sanctuary of *Bean There, Done That*, get some walking in, and hopefully, get acquired to the taste of coffee without sugar and milk. And water without apple Cordial/squash in it.

TRE seems a good idea. I'll set my daily window for 1-9 pm each day as I'm never hungry in the morning. I'll fast all day tomorrow. Think of it as a personal road-test. I'm expecting that exercise equipment I ordered over the weekend to arrive tomorrow. If I'm gonna bother putting in the burn I want to know I'm incinerating fat - as opposed to my time, effort, expectations, and desire to continue.

Now, the mathematicians among you will have figured out how long this fast I'm about to undertake *really* is. If I haven't eaten anything since my yogurt at 8:00 pm, eat nothing tomorrow, and then have my *first* bite to eat at lunch on Tuesday at 1 pm… that's a *41-hour fast*.

I'll write about it if I'm still alive this time tomorrow.

Calories Consumed:

Tuna = 120

Apple = 80c

Jacket Potato = 250

Yogurt = 55

~~Banana = 100~~

3 x Coffee = 150

3 x Squash = 60

Grand Total: 720

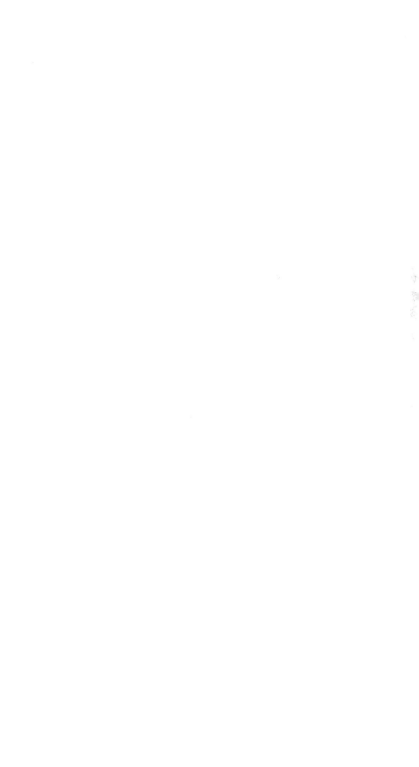

Day 8, or:
"A Full Day, Not Belly"

"I once told a girl I was Kevin Costner,
and it worked because I believed it."
- Saul Goodman, *Breaking Bad (2008-2013)*

<u>*Monday, July 1st, 2019*</u>

I haven't eaten for twenty-six hours.

It's two minutes after midnight as I type this, so (technically) I'm into day nine. Let me put this in perspective for you (and by "you" I mean *you*, Andrew, not anyone else. One day you're going to re-read all this and remind yourself of what you went through).

I'll go to bed around 2 or 3 am and wake up around 11 am as usual. I'll have a black coffee and a cigarette - or three - during my first hour being awake. I'll inevitably listen to the radio and do my morning ritual of checking my book royalties and ad spend and revenue. Then, around midday or so, I'll drive to *Bean There, Done That*. Unlucky Number 8 will probably be there, I'll have a black Americano (yes, *black* - more on that in a moment) and then drive home, take *The Lazy Route* to the fifth floor and

131

then have lunch. I anticipate this will occur around 1:15 pm, or thereabouts. So, all-in-all, I'll have fasted for just over 41 hours. That's almost two days.

You have to bear in mind that you're reading words typed by fingers attached to a hand an arm of a body that generally doesn't go without food for more than a couple of hours.

Now, to the question you're probably dying to know - how do I feel? More pertinently still, am I hungry? Respectively, the answers are: *great*, *thanks for asking*, and *absolutely not*.

I'm not hungry at all. I was told to expect a spike (or "pang" as we Brits say) of hunger around the times I am accustomed to eating, namely 2 pm and 8 pm. On *both* occasions I might have had a twinge of hunger. I barely noticed them.

I spent most of the day more alert and aware than I've ever been. Driving was easy and, dare I say, *safer* as a result? It's hard to tell, to be honest, but it sure felt that way. I didn't even crave food. I've not felt this good in a long, long time.

But at what price? If there's one to pay, I guess we'll find out soon.

Fasting is way, way easier than you think it is, Andrew. My recommendation to aid the process is two simple things:

1: Go about your day *as if* you've been eating. **Fool Yourself.** Busy yourself with the things you usually do. Counterbalance the extraordinary (lack of food) with the ordinary (work, daydreaming), in that respect, and…

2: If you do feel hunger, ignore it. Drink a glass of water to make it go away. I have a feeling the next time I crave dessert after a meal a simple glass of water might satiate that hunger. Kill it dead.

That said, here's what I *did* consume today.

- black coffee with a pinch of salt.

- green tea with a pinch of salt (sipping through a four-hour period this afternoon.)

- filtered water.

That's it.

I've had three coffees and two green teas since I woke up thirteen hours ago. I think I've had maybe three tall glasses of water. One of them was certainly when I woke up, and I have one on the go right now as I type. I must have had one during the afternoon, but I don't remember for sure.

Why did I fast?

To burn fat, apparently. Roughly six different sources on the subject of fasting I've read or watched have said that a sixteen-hour window is optimal - for beginners, at least. As ever, I'm pushing my own limit by going *nearly two damn days*. After sixteen hours (allegedly) your body starts to burn fat cells, which is the real key to weight loss.

They talk about the 16:8 approach in many of the online videos. 16 hours with no food, and an 8 hour window to eat whatever you like - within reason, of course. Not as difficult as it sounds if you don't like breakfast.

So, starting tomorrow - and all the way to my goal weight in three months' time - I've decided I'll eat *nicely* (that is to say, around 1200-1500 calories, but crucially, a massive reduction in refined sugar/carbohydrates and saturated fats) at once, and spend the next 22-23 hours fasting. In other words, I'm doing what I normally do; chilling out, sleep, drink coffee, etc.

If you have coffee and / or tea *with* milk (or creamer) you break your fast. If I wake up at 11 am and have a black coffee (with salt, which aids the brain's function in the absence of food, but it's not as bad as it sounds) then I *won't* have broken my fast.

Then, between 1 pm and 9 pm is my eight-hour window of potential food consumption. But I won't need eight hours because I'm blessed to not have to commute or work too hard. My window will be sensible and timed with my wife returning home. Maybe 7-9 pm.

I can do this.

Also, I can categorically say that you will not die if you fast. I'm not saying it'll be easy - especially if you *begin* your "project" or "diary" with a long fast after a heavy night of alcohol and a giant, sweaty kebab - but it can be done. I don't recommend you do *that*, so don't. It's something you need to build up to. At the very least, you should be on vague nodding terms with how it works and *why* you're doing it for it to work efficiently.

I walked into *Bean There, Done That* and noticed almost immediately that Unlucky Number 8 wasn't there. How very strange that this morbidly obese doorstop of a girl (for that is what she is) is not present at this - or any - time of day. Alas, I marched into the place of purveyance and approached the counter, knowing I was in for a tough time.

See, these guys know I take creamer with my Americano (black coffee). So I'm all geared up to stop them before they do it. That's the thing with baristas. They mean well. They're simply trying to be super-efficient, but there are some days you might want to change your order and they've gone way ahead of themselves.

There's one female barista manager who I'm on vague "hi" terms with. She's the manager at this particular branch. I'm asked if I want "the usual?" and I say, "Yes, but please don't put any milk in it today."

She looks at me as if I'm someone *different*. Ha. Give it another couple of months, my friend, and I will be. She asks why today of all days I've decided to go without milk. I explain I'm conducting an experiment…

"What? Like a diet?"

"Aww, nah," I huff, trying to play-down the D-Word. "It's more about the effect on the overall physique and mindset."

I hoped that the onslaught of words confused her, and it seemed to have worked a treat, judging by her baffled expression.

"Oh. Cool," came the confirmation.

I couldn't help but add a little spark of celebrity about it and (stupidly) went onto say, "Yeah, I'm writing a book about it."

"Oh. Are you?"

"Yep. Going well so far."

People are always impressed when you tell them you're an author. If you're a filmmaker (which I once was) the follow-up question is always "Oh, what kinda films? Are they adult videos? LOL!" (eye-roll, yeah, whatever) or they ask the *other* question, which is "Oh really? Have you made a film I might have seen?" to which the answer is invariably "no."

When you're an author, you never, ever, ever, *ever* get asked "Oh, have you written anything I might have read?" I refer specifically to people in polite society, such as in cafes. Baristas, checkout girls, the occasional sword-swallower, that kinda thing. I'm sure book convention attendees ask this question all the time. But in real, normal life? Never. Why is this? Here's my theory.

Nobody reads for pleasure, anymore.

With the advent of Prime Video, Netflix, picking loose hairs out of your scrotum, the *very last thing* people think to do is read for entertainment.

The chances are high that even *you* reading this book (and that includes you, Andrew, as *both* your chins know) eschew reading for binge-watching Netflix programs, or sitting through a film. Reading a book for fun is the last thing that enters your brains. It's one of life's little quandaries I have no intention of answering. Oh well.

A minute or two later, I'm sitting outside in my favorite spot by the window and chugging on the first of God-knows-how-many-cigarettes when a thought pierces my cranium like a sharp thing - "What if I ask the barista girl some questions for the book?" Has *she* noticed a change in me? I'm just over the halfway mark on this roller coaster. Is it too late? Enough of a drop to measure? Does she see me often enough? Does she even give a damn? What color panties is she wearing?

Much like the end of the last paragraph, I eventually talk myself out of the idea. It'll serve little purpose, anyway. I might well have changed my mind about this tomorrow and ask. But what exactly would I ask? I dunno yet. I'm rambling, now.

There's some very important stuff to get to.

Of all the eight days so far, today is the day I've learned the most - and not necessarily for the reasons you're suspecting.

Sure, I took *The Lazy Route* up the stairs. Oh, and my "gym" equipment came whilst I was out quaffing coffee like a stupid panda. Here's what I received.

1: *A Thigh Master.* Evidently made in China - and of weak plastic - but it appears to do the job. I suspect it'll break before this adventure is over.

2: *Two hand grips.* Better quality, and you can adjust the setting which means the spring moves out further. I have it set to the maximum (40kg) because my wrists (especially my right one) have always been strong due to excessive amounts of *<removed on editorial advice>*.

3: *A Power Bar.* Made by some narcissist in Japan, judging by the *Janglish* written on the box. "Most Powerful Superhuman Method", or some such nonsense. The Power Bar measures about two feet in length and bends in the middle. I doubt The Rock himself could bend it. It's rigid and tough. I *just about* managed to bend it by placing it on my stomach and burning every stored calorie I've consumed since February 1993 with my bare hands. I think I'll be using the Power Bar less often than the Thigh Master, to be honest. I quite like my limbs and want to keep them.

It's been going well. Intermittent bursts of fifty reps with each device is within my comfort zone. I'm enjoying them - particularly the first two devices I mentioned. I have to stress here that I am only using them to speed up the fat burning process. I have no interest in acquiring muscles. I just want to slim down and "be normal", to use the non-politically correct, staggeringly out of date vernacular of the day. Of course by "normal" I really mean "optimum weight for my height", and not some dribbling moron whose shoe size outnumbers his (or her, or its) IQ.

In short, I'm very sure I can take my coffee without milk and the smallest hint of sugar from now on. The amount of sugar I put in my coffee in the past was more of a placebo, now that I think about it for more than six seconds. I'm not kidding. The whole *Fool Yourself* methodology was in full force long before I started this thing - just as it is for *you*. I *think* I can survive on filtered water, now, too - and not have to add any apple Cordial/squash to it, which is less of a placebo because you can genuinely taste the apple with just a teardrop of the stuff put into the water. But when you're mostly resetting your taste buds as I've been doing so far, you notice the honest-to-goodness natural taste in food. At least, I hope that's the case when I consume something other than fish, potatoes, and fruit.

It took me a while to admit it but after every potato I've had so far I've actually managed to convince myself, especially in the first few days, that I had just eaten a kebab. Or a burger. That tin of tuna for lunch? A gorgeous ham and cheese sandwich with a domino-line of Texas BBQ-flavored Pringles. I was doing just that not ten days ago. It works. I can fool myself.

"See that cup of black coffee right there?" I asked Amelia as we sat at an outside table at a different branch of *Bean There, Done That*. The end of my finger pointed to my third black-and-salted coffee of the day, "As far as I'm concerned, that *has* milk and sugar in it, like normal."

"Pfft. Nonsense," she blurted. "I don't believe it."

"Well, I *believe* it. That's all that matters."

I take another sip and, for a brief moment, acknowledge the sour, distinctly milk-and-sugar-less taste of a drink I usually love. My attention had been drawn to the reality of it being purely "black" and nothing else. Then, I swallowed, and it felt normal. Milk, sugar, *everything*.

"I'm sorry, no. I don't believe it at all," Amelia repeated.

"It's part of the whole ***Fool Yourself*** thing I was talking about—"

She shakes her head, and it's precisely *here* where we need to freeze frame whatever image you have in your mind's eye of this particular interlude.

Because *this* - right here - is the most important thing I have learned. Not just since I started this project, but in years.

See, I had always wondered why Amelia had taken a sort of despondent backseat approach to what I'm doing. She's usually enthusiastic about everything I do. Very supportive. I've made some major, life-changing decisions that have affected us both, and almost always for the better. But this? Attempting to reach my (#1) goal weight of 12st? Not so much. It had been baffling me since I announced it all on Saturday June 22nd, two days before I started.

Then, the chink in the armor cracked.

"You need to be careful," she instructed with little humor.

"What?"

We got talking. She told me that what I'm writing is bound to be read by people who could get triggered. Worse, those reading it might try to attempt what I'm doing and injure themselves.

"I wrote this book for me, first and foremost," I explained. "If someone else wants to buy it and read it, then that's on them."

It seemed a perfectly reasonable rationale in a British accent to me because I don't make a habit of lying to anyone *other* than police officers. If anything, I'm brutally honest, for better or (usually) worse. This book is for me, and me alone. If you are reading it, then… well done. But don't you dare try any of what you're reading on yourself. Remember your vow in the introduction. Yeah, don't think I've forgotten.

Okay, okay, I get it. What you *want* to do is read the whole book and get an idea of what the process is like and try it for yourself. But you, dear reader, and I, are different. Hey, we may be extremely alike. But you're different. It seems to be working *so far* for me… but it might not work for you.

But wait, it gets better…

"A range of people are going to be reading this, Andrew," Amelia continued. "And lemme tell you something. Some people may treat this topic differently to others. You don't know how people will respond. How sensitive they could be."

"How do you mean?"

"Some might find this a very controversial topic."

Amelia went onto explain that some people do indeed take this subject extremely seriously. I think I do, too. I'm not doing this for fun. Amelia spoke of an altogether different kind of *serious* I'd not considered until now. Certain individuals keep their diets, food consumption etc, to themselves and vow never to explain themselves to anyone, ever.

As it transpires, Amelia was no different to those people.

"What?" I asked. "You mean to tell me that you've done the same?"

"Yep."

I admit that this came as something of a shock. I had to draw something out by way of a carefully-calibrated question. All the dialog is paraphrased, of course.

"Okay, if you were me, and you'd been doing all this, is there something you wouldn't reveal to me about it? Kept hidden?"

"Yes."

I didn't get much further than that. I didn't need an exact answer, but it sure as hell explained a lot about my and my wife's approach to food over the years. Amelia takes this subject *very* seriously - and with good reason.

We visited a local supermarket and, by pure chance, drove right past our regular Chinese takeout. I asked her what she wanted for dinner tonight. She said she hadn't decided just yet.

I pulled the car up in the parking supermarket lot and said, quite innocently, "If you want a Chinese, we can get one. It's right down the road."

She turned to me with an abruptness I'd never seen before and said, "Don't tell me what to eat."

We entered the store. Me, on an empty stomach, and her with a mission to procure some of her favorite foods. The hunt proved mostly fruitless We headed for the Chinese takeout place.

As we walked in, I half-suspected my sense of smell to go into overdrive and batter my stomach. In Britain our Chinese takeout places are often fish and chips shops, too. They cook and serve both. Inside, the waft of chips rifled up my nostrils - but never rung my hunger bell. A few seconds later, I caught a whiff of what I believe was crispy chili beef, but it might not have been because it's my favorite Chinese dish and my brain was probably taking cues from my morals and lying to me.

Then, I couldn't smell anything at all. Nothing. Any and all aromas just vanished, leaving me none-the-hungrier. That was at precisely the twenty-four hour mark of my fast.

We got home, and Amelia ate a couple of feet behind me (I must stress that she was on the sofa and I was at my desk. I don't mean she was deliberately two feet behind me, scoffing her dinner behind my back in some bizarre experiment.) I can't deny there was an initial waft of *whatever she had* drifting around and teasing me but, much like the Chinese takeout itself, it dissipated.

Well, that's some mighty fine will power you're exercising there, boy! About half an hour later, she left the empty cartons on the kitchen counter. I couldn't help but bend down and sniff around the half-consumed rice and chicken. Wow, it smelled divine. I smiled at the fact that one day I'll be able to eat that stuff again. But I didn't salivate, and the temptation to just take a mouthful not only didn't *occur,* but wasn't in consideration whatsoever.

If only I applied this kind of willpower and dedication to my business. Perhaps I'd be a millionaire by now?

But, as Amelia said during our coffee break, it's all about one word: *control.* The reason why people start doing one thing with one goal, and end up furthering the whole thing until the original thing is but a distant glint in history. She's afraid that my desire to reach my target weight *could* - as it has done for so many others - lead to something more destructive.

There's an old tale I remember that might explain this, and it's funny. Ready?

"I used to view so much adult material over the years. It became an obsession. It got to the point where I could only be satisfied by looking at pictures of *fully-naked women.*"

Okay, a bit crude, but hopefully you get the point. We all do it on our lives, don't we? Take the Pringles thing. "Oh, I'll just have three or four," — What, *tubs?*

Or "I know I'm halfway through the finale of Breaking Bad. I know, I'll just watch *one more episode* and *definitely* go to bed."

Yeah, right.

The fact is that such a change in many directions (goals, bodyweight, approach, to name but three) could very well lead to something better, or worse. This is why setting a goal is important. As you know, my only goal is as simple as it gets. I just want to reach my regular, healthy body weight of 12 stone (167 lbs / 76 kg). I want to do it by my 41st birthday. That's all. It takes two seconds to write down somewhere, which I've done *multiple times right here in this diary.*

I stand to reduce the risk of getting type 2 diabetes and other things just waiting to find a crack in my health armor. I need to be more active and healthier. I know at least one day of fasting already brightens my mood and makes me feel better. Active body, active mind. Maybe I'll write my own Harry Potter and become a multi-millionaire next year. Maybe that won't have happened because I *didn't* have a kebab the night before that gave me the germ of the idea.

You need a goal.

I thought until today that mine was to lose weight. I was wrong. My goal is to *lose fat*. Why? Because it's the fastest and most reliable route to getting to 12st within a reasonable time frame.

I'll leave you with this final thought…

What's your goal?

Calories Consumed:

Grand Total: 0

Day 9, or:
"Memento"

"Oh, God, Ted. I'm so hungry.
There's no chance I couldn't die, could I? From the hunger?"
- Fr. Dougal McGuire, *Father Ted* (1995)

<u>Tuesday, July 2nd, 2019</u>

I actually went forty-eight hours without food, and not forty-one as I had anticipated. I ate at 8pm tonight. Why forty-eight hours and not forty-one? There are two reasons why…

1: I wasn't hungry at all during that forty-eight hour period. Even today, the second day. You may remember I planned to eat around lunchtime. It wasn't necessary. How I feel right now as I type will explain this answer, which I'll do once I've explained…

2: Forty-eight hours is two days. I know what I'm like. If I had caved it at the forty-first hour, I'd have felt like a failure. I realize now that it's *precisely* this mode of thinking that could precipitate the kind of dangers Amelia spoke of yesterday.

Back to point #1, though, because it's important. One thing I am very good at is research. Being a full-time author means you have no choice. It's not about the quantity of research, but the *quality*. The only way you can truly get quality research is from deriving your information with a healthy dose of skepticism (obviously Rome is the capital of Italy - you don't need to research too far on that one). When it comes to methods - be it about pedagogy (teaching), nutrition, fire-eating methods, etc - you must ensure veracity. If you don't, it could harm or kill you. At least the last example would eliminate your halitosis for good, I guess. Talk about a five-hundred-pound solution to a five-pound problem, eh?

I've researched no fewer than twenty online videos and at least ten times as many journals, essays, and general information on websites such as the NHS. I was led to believe that fasting would make me more alert, and that drinking water would satiate the initial hunger pains.

The practical results for me?

YMMV (Your Mileage May Vary) but, for me, it's worked way better than anticipated. I salivated copiously during the first few days in between tuna and potatoes. Now I know why. My body absorbed food - way less than it was used to - and craved food more, hence the bouts of spitting. I didn't salivate at all whilst fasting, in the same way you *don't* salivate when you skip breakfast and lunch at work.

It all makes sense now.

One of my vows in the introduction specified that I wouldn't revisit old diary entries in this journal. I want to capture the truth; the evolution of my actions, and resulting mood and mental and physical performance. A brutally honest record of my thinking; how I felt, and my decisions to change things (if there were any).

I started this adventure because of the two things I outlined in the introduction. Tuna and potato.

I now realize I have made a huge mistake. Tuna is perfectly fine, but I'd have been better off with salmon. Potatoes are high in carbs, though not much else. I could have reset my taste buds and shrunk my stomach in a far more effective way.

Now, my thinking as I type this sentence at 11:38 pm on Tuesday, is that everything is essentially okay. There is light at the end of this ravenous tunnel. It's all over this coming Monday, so I will stick to the food intake plan as advertised. After all, what's a little high carb in relation to a lifetime of subsisting on McDonalds, Burger King, KFC, and all the good time?

Today's entry is going to work backwards. From right now as I type, and all the way back to when I woke up. Let's call it the *Memento* chapter (for all you Christopher Nolan fans out there).

Right now, some three or so hours after I ate, I am *really, really* hungry. It's gotten to the point where - yes - I'm salivating almost every second. I'm swallowing it all back, cautiously praying that saliva doesn't contain any high carbs or sugar. I know that sounds like a joke, but right now my own ability to ***Fool Yourself*** is starting to *work against me*. I know saliva doesn't contain anything at all but it feels like it does. It feels like I'm drinking lukewarm, saturated sugar extract.

At exactly 8 pm, just after my shower, I had my regular tin of tuna and *half* an apple. This time, I didn't add any Cayenne powder and no black pepper. It tasted like it always did. Actually, the tuna tasted terrific; so juicy and tender and lean, and full of flavor. I've decided I don't need the condiment additions, anymore. Why? Because this time last week I was adding a blob of full-fat creamer and sugar in my coffee. Today, I had no milk and *added salt, for goodness' sake!*

So, the taste bud reset is working for sure. I have a glass of water with apple squash on the go, as well. Now, it tastes like regular filtered water. The added flavor isn't making much of a difference. I know I can do straight-up filtered water. During my two-day fast I downed *at least* five glasses per day with relative ease.

It occurs to me now that it isn't really my taste buds that are resetting; it's that area of my brain *processing flavor* that is resetting. I'm no scientist (as you know) but I find it helps to think of it along those lines. Oh, hello again, Mr. ***Fool Yourself!*** If you truly believe you are drinking soda when you're really drinking water, then what's the difference?

I guess one could, in theory, extend the idea outside of food consumption. You *think* you're in love with your spouse? You think you're ill, when really it's mild hypochondria? If enough people tell Angelina Jolie that she's ugly do you think she'll believe it? I dunno. This is a whole metaphorical bargain bucket I don't really want to get into here. I'd much rather tuck into a mayo chicken from the fine establishment with the golden arches - and, *no*, before you ask - I'm *not* kidding.

From the moment I tossed the tuna tin in the trash, I began to crave mayo chicken burgers for some reason. I keep thinking about food. It probably goes without saying that I am counting the days until Monday, July 8th - *Kebab Monday*. Beautiful, long strips of lamb meat all criss-crossing over each other on a bed of soggy French fries (we call them chips in the UK), drenched in garlic mayo and chili sauce. Ugh, I think I'm going out of my mind. At least typing and focusing on relaying my thoughts is taking my mind off of it. For now.

Prior to dinner, or should I say "break fast" lol (now we know where the term came from!), I took a shower. Now, what I'm about to tell you could have something to do with eight days of dieting. But... I firmly believe I have lost more weight fasting than I have... well, *ever*.

Running my hands around my soapy legs was the first giveaway. Soaping a particular part of my body too disgusting to mention was much easier than it's ever been. The towels wrapped further around my thighs. The sides of my enormous gut (you know what I mean, the part above the love handles) have all but sunk in. I'm *tightening*. My curves are forming right angles and straight lines, as they ought to for most red-blooded men of a particular pulchritude. No further confirmation was needed than when I exited the shower and walked past Amelia. She looked me over, felt around my body, and finally acknowledged - for the first time since I began - that *something* was happening. I breathed a sigh of relief. She noticed my earlobes (of all places) were thinner, and smaller. A quick hug (genuine, not for the purposes of this journal) confirmed also that things had, indeed, tightened.

I can see it in my face, too. My boyish, good-looks have always contributed to me looking *somewhat* younger than I really am. I think the subtle chubbiness in my face took care of a lot of the legwork, anyway. But my double chin is swallowing back into my soon-to-be chiseled jawline. If I tuck my chin back to force a double chin effect, it's still there. But "normal" posturing with my head, and it's definitely gone.

Prior to the shower, Amelia and I visited a larger supermarket to get some more apples. We had a quick look at some of the foods I'll be eating once this *fortnightmare* (for that is what it's become, for reasons I'll go into, below) is over. Next Monday is the now-famous Kebab Monday. I am *seriously* considering fasting for three days next week. Tuesday, Wednesday, and Thursday. I miss the feeling of alertness, keenness, and, as long as I return to eating, I'm going to be salivating - and that HAS to stop.

Among some of the potential dinners I could be having, one lights up my eyes. I could have a potato with baked beans and a modest amount of cheese. Potato flirts dangerously with carb levels, but that's okay. Beans are high in fiber, so that's good. And cheese in moderation is good for the skin and other minerals such as calcium, which is good for my bones. Beans and cheese is an orgasm for the mouth belonging to the body whose hands are typing this very sentence. Ugh, what I wouldn't give for just a spoonful right now. With my taste buds all "vanilla'd" it'd probably taste like pure sex (the good kind - not the creepy, sleazy kind).

I'll create a proper hit list for dinners later. Have you noticed I've not mentioned lunches? Okay, let me breakdown my revised plan for you. As of Tuesday next week (or, if I *do* fast for three days, then Thursday at 8pm) here's my plan in perpetuity until I reach my goal weight of 12st by my 41st birthday in October.

1: Intermittent fasting begins *now*. Because I work from home, I can afford to eat one meal per day. 8 pm. I'll scoff all my carbs, fats, sugars, nutrients, you name it. *A one-hour feeding window.* Why? Because it means I'll be on a 23:1 regime. A one-hour window to eat, followed by a twenty-three hour fasting window to burn fat. Because the fat burning process occurs at the sixteenth hour, I'll enjoy about seven hours of *real burn*, not to mention the longer-term effects of my body burning sugar instead of other stuff I don't need to burn.

2: SUGAR IS THE ENEMY. Sorry, let me repeat this. NO MORE SUGAR. Why? It's poison. Sugar converts to fat, and is stored in the body to burn up when you aren't eating anything. Like the cavemen did back in 1955 (ho-ho!) when they hunted for food for days and days without eating. The body burned fat to keep them alive. Guess what? That's what I want *until* such time as I reach my goal weight of 12st. Once I hit it, I'll go regular. Now look, I'm not stupid. Well, actually I am, but…

Whatever. The fact is that one *cannot avoid* fat entirely. But I *can* avoid putting less of it in me, and the less I put in, the less effort my organs have to burn it off *and* stop all that poisonous sugar being flung through my veins and crashing into my limbs to cause amputations, or up to my eyes to cause blindness.

3: VERY FEW CARBS. Especially refined carbs. Imagine a parking lot with an entrance barrier. All those spaces in the parking lot are pockets within your body, filling up with fat once the liver has turned sugar into fat. When those spaces (or "stores") fill up, you get "titch bits", for example. Or love handles. Or a big belly. So, we need to burn them away, right? Now, imagine the barrier preventing access is *insulin*. Every time you eat carbohydrates, the barrier closes (i.e. your insulin goes up). In order to burn the fat in the parking spaces, we need access to them in those parking spaces. But the barrier is down. And carbohydrates are the barrier, in this silly analogy of mine. We need to batter that barrier away to open up the path so we can get in and burn the fat. So, less carbs/insulin is the answer. Go ahead, body! The barrier has gone - *now get burning*. It's really that simple. If we don't burn fat, we stay fat. A bit like if you *don't* burn Adolf Hitler to death in an incinerator, then he'll remain unburned and very much alive until we do.

In Summary:

- a 23:1 hour intermittent fasting window. For the 23 hour period I can only drink pure black coffee, pure green tea, and filtered water. But, hey, during that one hour period? I can guzzle down as many coffees with cream as I want. Not that I will, of course.

- Said one-hour window occurs between 8-9 pm because my wife gets home and we can cook and eat.

- Drink *filtered* water as and when I feel hungry.

- Exercise (such as it is!) as usual. Move as usual. The body will burn fat with minimal movement, but more with some encouragement.

- Cut sugar and carbs out as much as I can. Once I'm at goal weight, I know I could, theoretically, eat sixteen Big Macs and wash it down with a large regular soda. Why? Because I could then *fast* for a while and burn it right off. The bonus of that would be I *won't* be a fat lump of lard when that happens, and so shifting the weight should be relatively easy - particularly when I'm used to fasting.

If you'd have told me that I would be meditating this time last week, I wouldn't have believed you - and indeed it wasn't the case. But today I did. I meditated in my own way at about 3pm. Total zen-like paralysis, right in the middle of my fast. It was absolutely serene. I'm not a proponent of mythical creatures and wacky, Eastern philosophies, but it worked. I don't really like to think of it as meditation - more an extreme "chill". The problem with calling it that is because one's use of the word "chill" is one rung up the ladder of being an annoying a-hole, and a sidestep towards being a hipster, and it's a well-known fact that hipsters (as a general rule) must to be hung, drawn, and quartered and have their stupid beards scalped off their faces by hanging their puny bodies from the nearest - and highest - available bridge at the earliest opportunity.

So, rather than "chill", I'll go with the term "extreme-do-whatever-it-is-that-you-do-to-relax". Yep, I can see that term catching on. The point is, it's awesome. Find yours and try it out. Heck, you don't need me for this; the chances are good that you're already doing it, anyway. For me, it was listening to Strauss' *Blue Danube Waltz* with my feet extended from my desk chair and my eyes closed. I do all three of those things all the time - usually two at a time - so entering that med state was a piece of… no, *don't say it*. Mmmmm… all spongy and warm, drizzled in chocolate, like Belgian fudge…

I need a cigarette. I'll be back in a second, don't go anywhere.

Ahh, that's better. See, cigarettes are an appetite suppressor. I'm still hungry, though.

At 2:30 pm, I shit in my pants.

Hold on, let me explain. I walked onto the balcony with a cigarette in my mouth and let out what I *thought* was going to be a little fart. Sure enough, some gas came out, but very little in comparison to the squelchy, wet feeling that followed. Fortunately, *the majority* of it didn't escape (my now significantly reduced) butt cheeks. So, it was with a modest amount of trepidation that I penguin-walked on my heels to the bathroom and set about surveying the damage. Pants down, I assess the result. To call it *feces* is probably inaccurate; it was more like brown water.

Around midday, I went to the bathroom to try and empty my bowels… to discover, of course, that they were empty. A day and a half of no food, and you'll be lucky to get a duck's quack from your pucker, let alone a decent stool. No *crap*, Sherlock, as they say.

I removed the offending garment by doing what *you* do in just such a situation; a futile attempt to remove my fricken feet through the leg holes of my pants *and underwear* without turning them inside-out as my shins rifle upwards.

Two minutes later, a fresh pair of underwear. The same ones I *wasn't* wearing when I was at…

Bean There, Done That, around 12:45 pm. Sitting on my own with my black coffee, I lifted the lid and sprinkled half a small packet of salt into it and stirred it around. The second day of my fast and everything was terrific. I felt a sense of calmness and serenity. Not much to report, here, apart from the fact that I've noticed Unlucky Number 8 *not* taking up three seats and the entire left-side of the façade for a while. It's been three, whole days, actually. What's happened to her? Did she eat herself out of existence?

Prior to that was the bathroom attempt I mentioned above.

Before that, I had the first coffee, and then cigarette, of the day. When that rolls around, I usually feel my bowels churning, ready for war with the porcelain. It didn't happen today, though.

Then, before that, I woke up. I wasn't hungry. I'd slept better than ever, I think. Apart from when I was a kid and life had yet to deal me any bad hands.

I'm getting really tired now. I've been typing for almost an hour. I blame having dinner for this. At midday tomorrow, that will have been sixteen hours of fasting, as I've mentioned, and I suspect the hunger will dissipate once again.

So, dear reader (Andrew), I'll leave you with my final thought for the day. Calories, calorie-counting, and a low calorie diet without fasting appears to me to be an utter waste of time.

We're not burning calories, here. We're burning *fat*. In other words, we're killing sugar and carbs as much as possible. So, that final calorie count at the end of each day is an utter waste of time, as far as I'm concerned.

I'll include today's count out of courtesy but starting tomorrow I don't think I'll bother. There's just no point in doing it. I may as well add how many couches I didn't sit on, too, for all the good it does.

Can you see how this journal has been beneficial? I have vowed to never, ever re-read or tamper with what I've written. This diary is meant to be raw and evolutionary... heck, potentially revolutionary. With the right support and medical advice if just *one* person reading this is inspired to change their ways for the better - and potentially reverse a fatal, forthcoming, or ongoing condition - then all of this would've been worth doing.

But, Andrew, this is for you. If you're doing this right and you sustain the weight loss, then at least you know you've won if you never have to read any of this ever again.

Calories Consumed:

Tuna = 120

Half an apple = 40

Water with added Apple squash x 3 = 10

Grand Total: 150

Day 10, or:
"Fat Man & the Beard"

"Mate, you're fat, and I'll throw you in the river."
- Ray Winstone, *Love, Honor & Obey (2000)*

<u>Wednesday, July 3rd, 2019</u>

It's probably pretty obvious to you, dear reader, that I am not revisiting previous diary entries and adjusting them. I'm not in the business of fixing the past; only the future. Yes, I realize how pithy and faux-prophetic that last sentence sounds. It pained me just to write it.

I bring this up because only yesterday I decided to stop recording my calories. I realize this was something of a mistake. While I was writing last night I was incredibly hungry having just broken a 48-hour fast. I guess you could say my judgment was clouded but at the time I meant every word. I did some more research after last night's entry and readjusted my plan.

Simply put, I need to "up" my calorie intake if my body is to operate at a high metabolic rate to burn off the fat once it's run out of food to chew through. The sixteen-hour process. I've also decided that when we get to what I affectionately term "*the outtroduction*" I'll leave all the links to videos and periodicals I think are the best ones for you to digest, if you'll forgive the pun.

I reached something of a breakthrough after I wrote yesterday's diary entry. I decided to adjust my good-food-intake starting today, and with good justification.

It's my belief (and I can substantiate this with an anecdote you're going to read later in this chapter) that I have, indeed, shrunk my appetite after ten days. I have also reset my taste buds sufficiently enough. If yesterday's first bite of tuna after 48 hours was the trailer, then the movie would roll round later this evening, which it did.

You know as well as I do that I consumed around 800-900(ish) calories each day since Monday, June 24th. Sounds good, right? Wrong. I *should* have been controlling the amount of sugar and carbohydrates I put in my body, as they're more important.

My body has been burning 800 calories-worth of fuel each day which results in a slower metabolism. A lower metabolism means that when I'm fasting (and believe me, I'm skilled at it now!) my body is burning fat at a slower rate.

Solution? Keep my proposed 22:2 (hours not eating, black coffee, water etc, when I eat) window of fasting and consume more calories within that window. 800 calories just won't cut it. *I can be burning more fat, faster, if I up my calorie intake.*

So, instead of including today's calories at the end of this chapter, I'll include them here so you can see what I ate. You'll be surprised at some of it.

Ready?

Calories Consumed:

Artichokes / 1 x tin of tuna - 240

Jacket potato - 250

Reduced fat baked beans (1 x tin) - 300

Grated Mozzarella Cheese - 100

Banana - 100

3 x large organic strawberries - 50

Grand Total: 1040

For the "lolz" (ugh, please shoot me. My trying to be "hip" gets irritating) I took a photo of tonight's dinner. Jacket potatoes, smothered in low fat baked beans and a healthy sprinkle of Mozzarella. *Mmmmmmmmmmm.*

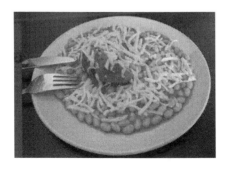

That's right, I "upped" my calorie intake. I won't go into the measurements (grams used etc) because it isn't worth it. If you try to do the same thing, you'll end up in a different store, buying different products, and it'll all get complicated.

I'm a firm believer that there are three food duos that go together to create a palatable nirvana. Here they are:

1: Bananas and smoking cigarettes.

2: Milk chocolate and pure orange juice.

3: Full-fat baked beans (Heinz, etc) and grated cheddar cheese.

4: (Bonus non-food-related): Having sex on methamphetamine, $C_{10}H_{15}N$ (a.k.a "Speed").

If you've not tried any of the above you are seriously missing out on life (apart from #4 - please don't start all that). Most of the orgasms I've had in my life pale into insignificance when compared to any *one* of the above-mentioned items.

So, when I discovered that potatoes were okay (high carb, but what can you do?), and beans were high in fiber (I owe my toilet some messy assaults, lately) and certain types of cheese were okay to consume, I didn't need telling twice. Nor did I need convincing that I should change my food intake.

See, for most of the day, I was thinking "No, Andrew. Don't do that. You've already had the book cover made and it mentions a diet of tuna, fruit, and potatoes." For a while, there, I stopped myself.

Then, just before Amelia came home, I talked myself out of it. Hell, I *need* calories to burn, and there are only six days left of this diary to go.

So, why not change it up? Why not adjust and record what I'm doing before I run out of pages, so it benefits me when I inevitably re-read this book in the year 2035 when I've put all the weight back on?

Amelia and I went out and bought artichokes, low-fat beans, cheese - basically everything that had never appeared on my calorie hit list until today, and got back home around 7:15 pm.

Now, because I've been fasting for sixteen hours (yep, black coffee, green tea, salt, you know the drill) I wanted to practice having lean protein exactly one hour before my main meal.

So, I prepared a bed of artichoke (approximately one-third of the glass tub) and scooped out the tuna with a fork and made a kind of paella with it. A light dust of Cayenne and black pepper (purely for calorie purposes, you understand) and - BOOM! - one delicious starter.

I had never had artichokes in my life before today. How the hell did I *never* have artichokes? They're wonderful - and, get this, with tuna they're absolutely gorgeous.

They're also oilier than a oiled-up stripper on a dancing pole, though. The glass damn-near plummeted out of my palm a few times, and Amelia told me off for touching the cupboard doors, drawers, the floor, possibly even the ceiling, with my grubby, greasy hands. I could have sworn I cleaned up after myself but - as a married man - clearly my hygiene standards can't possibly compete with a woman far superior to me in every single way with absolutely no exceptions.

Hang on, Andrew, I hear you ask. Why artichokes?

I discovered that when you're breaking a *prolonged* fast (i.e. 24+ hours) that you should really eat a bit of lean protein and preferably some plants, and in particular, artichokes, because they aid the process of reintroducing your stomach to food. There's science behind it, which you'll inevitably stumble upon in the links at the end of the book. I'm not a scientist, as you know.

Then, you eat your main meal about an hour after that.

I swore blind to you in the introduction (Vow #1) that I wouldn't get scientific because, let's face it, none of us are good at maths or science these days. It's actually a statistic that college graduates are more qualified to *make a documentary* about science and maths than actually *do* either of those subjects. Why is this? I think it's because everyone wants to be in the media, for some reason. I'm no different. You're probably not, either - but it doesn't help us get rid of those "titch bits", does it?

You need to think forward *a lot* during this process and avoid a reluctance to adapt. I'm speaking well ahead of myself because this could all backfire quite spectacularly. Indeed, a part of me (and Amelia) wondered if, when I consumed this abnormally large quantity of food / calories in such a short time span, that I might get sick, or worse, explode - like that angry dude in *Big Trouble in Little China*.

Well, here's the thing. Thinking ahead - when I hit my goal weight, my sophomore goal is to *keep the damn weight off, thankyouverymuch*. Preferably until the end of recorded time or when I die, whichever is the sooner.

So, I've decided that my long-term, everyday-slimline-Andrew will be consuming 1,500 calories per day, and preferably once-a-day at around dinnertime, in order to get that wonderful 22:2 intermittent fasting ratio going on.

Of course, some days (and I do mean days) I might go out for a cooked breakfast, or stuck on a ten-hour flight, or holed up in an interrogation room being questioned by the police about something I never did, or whatever, and that'll be my fasting plans well and truly screwed. But those days are rare.

That's the plan.

Listen up, Mr. Mackay. From now till your 41st birthday, your fat ass is on a strict 1,200 calories per day for dinner - and two hours to eat it. Do you understand what you're reading? Does that little voice in your head that speaks when you read a book come across loud and clear? You want chocolate? Tough. You want that McDonald's breakfast? No, I'm afraid not. You can have those things when you reach your goal weight and not before. Oh, and when you *do* have them, well, you're going to be intermittent fasting anyway, so it probably won't make much of a difference. You can burn it off rather easily with a fast.

Tomorrow I'm going to have exactly the same dinner again, but *two* potatoes instead of one. Why? An extra 250 calories to bump my total into the 1,200s where I should be; the optimum calorie count deficit to get my body burning fat for the next twenty four hours. Between eight and twelve of those hours my body will burn the food (or more specifically the nutrients and make-up of the food, the food itself will turn to brown sludge and greet me the following day in the bathroom) but… when it runs out, it'll have a further six-to-eight hours to continue burning *at the same speed* and start getting around to all that damn fat.

Lesson ends.

Now, the interesting bit…

By the time I had my artichoke and tuna medley, I was absolutely stuffed. It was tasty and filling. An hour later, I had the potato and beans and cheese. Now, by the end of *that*, I was *really, really* fit to burst. I felt like I had undone the previous ten days and blasted my way back up to 217 lbs / 15.5 stone. And *then* I had the banana and three strawberries.

Psychologically, this might have smashed anyone else's journey to pieces. For me, though, it didn't because I now know *why* I am eating what I'm eating.

Do you, reader, know *why* you eat?

Food for thought… *probably quite literally*.

While I was sitting outside *Bean There, Done That* at around 1 pm, drinking my salty coffee, I… oh, wait, I forgot to tell you. Amelia and I bought Pink Himalayan salt today. A finer, richer, more effective salt to add to my coffee / green tea to aid the fasting process. Sorry, I can't be bothered to rewrite this paragraph. I've only just thought of it.

Where was I?

Oh yeah. Today while I was having my coffee I found myself turning off the radio and just watching people. I absorbed the ambiance as the shareholders of Marlboro rubbed their hands at the skyrocketing stock value due to how many cigarettes I was chugging through.

An extremely overweight guy around my age came and sat uncomfortably close to me on a neighboring table. Like, he was really close. If he so much as sneezed, the side of his right man-breast would have kissed my shoulder. I didn't move away because I couldn't. Instead of kicking up a mini-fuss (he had three other tables to choose from, after all) I stared at him and watched what he was doing. It was lunchtime, and he was facing in the other direction.

He'd chosen a cold chocolate drink *thing* - no doubt ending with "cino" - in a clear, plastic cup with a useless paper straw designed to disintegrate like soggy toilet paper the instant you clamp your lips around the end. For lunch, he had a baguette bought in the store; some white meat filling which was probably chicken and a white sauce which was hopefully mayonnaise. And lettuce, let's not forget the lettuce. He had a packet of crisps, but I couldn't see which flavor it was, not that I gave a damn. Crisps are crisps, no matter which way you slice them.

And so it was that this dude chomped away like someone who had found a time-traveling machine, walked into Barnes & Noble, found a book called *The Hunger Diaries*, clocked the name of the author, figured out where this branch of *Bean There* was and what time I'd be there, traveled back in time, and deliberately sat stupidly close to me *to eat his fricken lunch while I was fasting with nothing but a tin of tuna and half an apple in my system.*

I'm over-dramatizing, of course. It's my job. I make my living from doing just that. But... I caught his face in profile and noticed that he had facial hair. Specifically, facial hair that ran under his chin and above his neck. More specifically, a *beard*.

Something in my brain clicked and spat out a deeply-held belief that - until today - had no reason to unearth itself.

What you're about to read next could well be extremely uncomfortable - especially for male readers - but you've read this far so I assume you're totally cool with my bizarre outlook on life - *unless you've accidentally opened the book at this page, in which case, STOP READING and go back to the beginning. You're not ready for this bit, yet. You need to make your vow, for one thing. Go back and we'll see you here, shortly.*

As for the rest of you... are you ready to hear this insane belief I hold after forty years on this planet? Please don't hate me. It's just an observation, and today I backed it up with wildly insufficient data.

But, anyway. Here we go.

<u>Fat men have beards to disguise their fat faces.</u>

OUCH-O-RAMA!

I think I deserve a Nobel Prize, or something.

I have a sneaking suspicion that we all know this, though. Hell, you should conduct the following experiment yourself, just so you know I'm not going mad. What I'm about to tell you is nothing particularly new; the fat dudes *certainly* know it (and I'm still one of them, sadly), and so do the girls. In fact, it's *so* obvious to others that shaving their facial hair off and prancing around with a giant neon sign above their heads reading "*I AM FAT!*" would be less blatant.

Not *all* men who have a beard, or a goatee, are fat, of course. It's a bit like what they say about terrorists - but we can change that up. *Not all bearded men are obese, but all obese men are bearded.*

Wait. Before you run off and tell everyone I've compared obese people to suicide bombers, just think about what I've told you for one second. I *haven't* said what you think I've said. Get it in context.

I realize it's a ridiculously and desperately unfair thing to have said. Further, it's bound to be statistically inaccurate. So, me being me - a staunch proponent of research - I decided to *count all these obese dudes* walking past my table for a twenty-minute period. I would have counted the obese women, too, but few of them have beards.

Hundreds of pedestrians walk past in all directions every hour as I sit outside *Bean There, Done That*. I ran (waddled) back into the store and asked for a napkin (because *Bean There* hides them due to patrons stealing them by the pack) and a pen. The bearded, fat-averse barista gave me a napkin and a pen, and I panted and wheezed back to my table.

For the next twenty minutes I checked off (in multiples of five, like a prisoner counting the days in his cell) the following:

1: LEFT column: Every time I saw a *man* I considered to be significantly overweight and / or obese.

2: RIGHT column: Every time one of those men had enough facial hair to cover their flabby chin / neck.

That's it.

From 1:10 pm to 1:30 pm - here are the results.

- Overweight / Obese men = 60

- of which had a beard = 42

Wow. Are you seriously telling me that forty-two hideously overweight men out of sixty have a beard?! The results shocked me. That's well over half; getting on for 75%. I could work out the exact percentage. Actually that's an utter lie. I can't work out the percentage without Google, and I'm on a roll, here, and I don't want to minimize Scrivener. Besides, this explanation is funnier and more revealing. Leave me alone.

The result makes total sense to me. I realize the sample study is not statistically significant or anywhere near the kind of quality *Ipsos Moron* conducts, but what I *can tell you* is that I counted sixty individual obese men over a twenty-minute period like a very inconspicuous hawk… *and forty-two of them had beards.*

I haven't quite figured out what this actually means, though. Well, not entirely. If I let my prejudices run wild I could cook up a theory which will at least get you thinking, which I'll do in a few seconds. It certainly says something about my quiet hometown of Chrome Valley that *two* dangerously overweight men walk past where I'm sitting every minute.

So, here's my theory.

Those significantly overweight / obese men *might* (and I do stress that term "might", for sake of debate) sport beards because:

1: They are in denial, which can only mean…

2: It works for them.

They're fooling nobody, of course. You think obfuscating your double / triple / quadruple chin renders you thinner-looking to others? In my eyes it makes you look more grizzly, like a big, fat bear. I'm often asked "Does this dress make me look fat?" to which the reply I keep in my head is "No, your face does."

Thus, we can only deduce that they're fooling themselves. In other words (yep, you're way ahead of me) they are enacting my soon-to-be-patented **Fool Yourself** ideology. And stone me if that isn't the very crux of the ideology of this book, and the very skill - for that is what it is - one needs in order to shed weight.

Let that sink in for a moment.

I also forgot to mention something else. Around 7 pm, when Amelia and I were walking back to our car with our groceries, we saw a dangerously overweight girl sitting on a bench in an enclave on the pathway. She had one tree-chunk of a leg resting on a chair. She looked desperately unhappy. It's possible she'd just got done crying. It was our friend, Unlucky Number 8, no doubt maximizing her time away from home even though *Bean There, Done That* had closed for the day. A part of me (the flabby part, probably) felt a bit sorry for her. That part of me quickly blushed and climbed out of sight. Put simply, it's not until she sorts herself out that she'll be truly happy.

I've given all this a bit of thought. I think I've come across as something of what the left-field thinkers call a "fat shamer." That certainly isn't my intention. I'm fat myself. Is it possible for a fat person to be a fat shamer? That'd be like a Nazi general accusing Heinrich Himmler of being right-wing. Wait, no, no, don't take that Nazi analogy seriously. It's a *joke*.

Fun Fact: Himmler was also born on my birthday (but in a very different year). Simon Cowell was born on the exact same day, too. Connection? *#ConspiracyTheory*.

Instead of getting all annoyed about jokes, why don't we get all upset about the insurmountable strain our healthcare system is experiencing because of our rising obesity epidemic? You know, stuff that actually *matters*. Why not get your placard rewritten from "XYZ jokes offend me" to "Free health care for all!" or "No More Cuts to the NHS!"?

Amelia told me in no uncertain terms today that she'd rather I just *tell* her what I want, rather than why I want it. "Oh, I wanna get some artichokes because—" quickly got cut off with a response along the lines of "Yeah, whatever. Let's get them."

This leads me to my final thought of the day. If you choose to do something like this, then remember these two things, because they are true. Oh, don't get me wrong, I *know* you *think* these things won't apply to you. Guess what? *They will.* Anyway, here are the two rules you'd be a fool to ignore or not take seriously:

1: Don't expect anyone (especially those close to you) to take as much of an interest in your fat-burning "quest" as you do.

2: Certainly *do not impose* on others about it. Keep your mouth shut.

And this, dear reader, is why I chose to tell no one about this little endeavor (see vow #6.) The only reason Amelia is kept updated is because it's impossible to hide it from her. But I've not told my mom. Or any of my friends.

This last part is important for two reasons. I realize I'm dumping a lot of info on you but, soak it up and let it ferment.

Reasons why telling nobody about your weight loss *thing* is a good idea:

1: You won't get bombarded with phone calls and messages asking how it's going.

2: There will be no naysayers or people who tell you it can't be done.

3: If you leave a long enough period, you can conduct a test. You were fat the last time they saw you. The next time you see them? *Say nothing.* Let them volunteer the revelation. "Hang on, have you lost weight!?" - and then you know it's working.

As it happens, the last day of this diary will be "Kebab Monday" (July 8th) when our cleaner - whom I shall call Beryl - comes for her once-a-month cleaning of our apartment. She hasn't seen me since the first Thursday of June - well before I started all this. I'll say nothing, of course, and act normal. If she says anything I'll make sure I record it for you.

Okay, this chapter has gone on long enough. Since you didn't ask, I am *still* not hungry after my higher-calorie dinner tonight. I'm sipping water and keeping hydrated because I genuinely want to walk the two miles to *Bean There, Done That* tomorrow.

One last thing before I tell you about stuff getting bigger. When I finished my shower, I stupidly managed to walk hip-first into the door handle in the front room. That event hurt, but wasn't terribly significant. What *was* significant is that, on the rebound, I manage to cut through the skin on a jagged edge of the housing that traps the bolt on the door frame. It bled quite a bit. Was this down to a reduction of food? Amelia put a band aid on it. I'm sure it'll be fine.

And finally… *stuff that gets bigger.*

My glasses keep slipping down my *fricken face*. Pushing them the bridge of my nose is a constant struggle. My skin isn't wet, or oily, and I'm not sweating. Amelia told me my earlobes are thinner, as you may remember.

But get this. My shoes are getting bigger, too. When I wash my hands, my fingers have slimmed down, as well as my wrists. It feels like I'm giving a midget a manicure. And, lastly, my pants (UK version: trousers) have outgrown my waist somewhat.

I wear light linen pants (trousers) during the summer. They have a zip, buckle, and two cotton strings that tie together. Even with the strings tied *very* securely, they're slipping down, now…

Right. Now I'm off to watch Morgan Spurlock's *Super Size Me* for the umpteenth time. It's required viewing for this sort of thing.

After that I shall go to bed and *not* enact vow #7.

Yeah, you're gonna have to flip back to the introduction to remind yourself what that vow was about (lol!) - what can I say? I'm mean like that.

Goodnight.

Day 11, or:
"Who Are You, and What Have You Done with My Husband?"

"Brothers are gettin' it together, and if you ain't part of the solution, man, you're part of the problem."
- Willie, *Born on the 4th of July (1989)*

<u>Thursday, July 4th, 2019</u>

A very happy 4th of July to all my American readers, and I mean that very, very sincerely. It's been 243 years since you took leave of us unwieldy Brits and set about conquering the world on your own terms.

The result of this - at least latterly - is that we in the UK are now taking the North America's lead on a few things. Our NHS is destined, sadly, to no longer be free at the point of service. I'm fully expecting us to move to an insurance model, like you have. Us Brits already know what I'm about to type but, in case you don't know, we don't have cash registers in hospitals. We pay for medical services with our taxes. When we have an accident, heart attack, accidental castration, or whatever, we get collected (for free) in an ambulance to a vastly understaffed, under-

183

appreciated, and over-stressed bunch of nurses and doctors on seventy-five-hour shifts without a break, thereby increasing our chances of dying from the tiniest of mistakes they make. And that's not to mention the sepsis and bacterial issues at hospitals we're having to dodge for fear of getting killed.

I bring this up because I glean from the news that obesity has now overtaken smoking as the #1 leading cause of preventable deaths, such as strokes, diabetes, and erectile dysfunction, to name but three, and close with one of the ruder examples I could think of for a cheap joke.

But it's *not* a joke, is it?

This is serious. Like our friends in the U.S., we're becoming increasingly tolerant of commercials on social media and peak-time TV for sugary drinks and fast food. The toys in the Happy Meals draw in the kids. It's much easier to grab a quick burger or foot-long sub than anything else, these days.

But do you know what's *really* fascinating?

Anyone who's too lazy to fix their issues is prime material to enact **Fool Yourself** and rectify everything. Nobody's too busy that they can't change their ways and *not* die eventually. Or have I got that wrong?

It's precisely these thoughts that ran through my head today as I *finally* walked the two miles to *Bean There, Done That*. It was an especially hot and sunny day, too. I decided I needed more exposure to the sun, though, so all was well.

The walk went well. I felt a lot lighter than I've previously experienced and managed the walk in just under 45 minutes. Three women smiled at me, two of whom I definitely *would*. The one I *wouldn't* was a lot older than me. The other two were probably just being polite. The point is that the smiles wouldn't have occurred when I was near-obese. I never made eye contact with anyone when I was out like a typical Brit. Eye contact is Kryptonite to us Londoners, and we never, ever do it, for fear of utter embarrassment. I found myself making eye contact and smiling with a great deal of politeness. Do you know how your new, favorite, cynical, still-overweight Amazon best-selling author felt when he did this?

He felt *great*.

Unlucky Number 8 wasn't at the coffee store today, once again. I presume she's still turning oxygen into carbon dioxide because Amelia and I saw her a couple days ago crying on a park bench. I do wonder what's happened to her. In my mind, she's finally succumbed to the will of her father and been grounded for being fat *and* failing to find a job within a reasonable delay. In truth, who even knows if that's even correct? She could be married with six children and a retired multi-millionaire for all I know.

Last night's meal of high fiber - particularly the beans - means I farted the small hours away last night before bed. This morning's dump thundered-in right on cue; around midday. And, boy, did it feel good to expunge that stuff through my anus and into the toilet bowl. I didn't break as much wind during my walk. I've had the same dinner once again tonight. This time, though, in order to bolster the calorie intake in a healthy way, I returned - for the first time since day one - to my mostly-uneaten cashew nuts. A full bag is 1,200 calories. I had about a third. You can do the math on the calorie count so I don't have to.

Calories Consumed:

Artichokes / 1 x tin of tuna - 240

Jacket potato - 250

Third of a bag of cashews - 300

Reduced fat baked beans (1 x tin) - 300

Grated Mozzarella Cheese - 100

Banana - 100

3 x large organic strawberries - 50

Grand Total: 1340 (Approx.)

It's now two-and-a-half hours since I ate dinner (it's 12:30 am as I write this sentence) so that means I'm part-way into my new decision I made today. I'm fasting for another 48 hours. "Why are you doing that *again*?" I don't hear you ask because you're too far away. And you didn't ask it in the first place; but now I've posited it you're definitely thinking it and so I'll give you the answer.

Honestly, I felt so great during the last fast that I want to do it again. I "upped" my calorie count today and yesterday in view of doing it, but now I've decided to go ahead and just do it.

I love the feeling of not being hungry and razor-sharp in my overall approach to life. I think it could even help me write my next book (it's a neo-psychedelic thriller called *Somnambulist*) which I plan to start writing next week.

Now, look. I really don't ever, ever, *ever* want to be *that guy*. You know the type. The annoying runt who quits smoking and then tells everyone about it and how they, too, should quit smoking. Or the a-hole who went on a fad diet and told everyone else to do the same. The high-and-mighty, high-falutin' hipster who's discovered a gluten-free, vegan planet in the Omega II multiverse and wants you to hop aboard the *StarShip Yawn* for an intergalactic adventure of planet-based tedium and sycophancy.

As Amelia drifted off to sleep, I told her I was embarking on another 48-hour fast - starting this very evening. She looked a bit worried, but it wasn't long before we started arguing about it. Then, a light bulb moment occurred to her.

What if she joined me?

Hmm. See, if this was you, I'd advise you to re-read the opening introduction and check out the rules and reasons for why you want to do it in the first place. I told her what to expect if she elected to try it. She'll be waking up a good 4-5 hours earlier than me. I need to keep my body clock stable (rise at 11 am, sleep at 3 am) at least until I finish this journal. So, I gave her some tips. I told her about the coffee / salt, green tea, and filtered water thing. She's not especially good at the whole **Fool Yourself** thing in many respects. In certain areas she's an absolute master of self-control but, in this instance of having her food schedule tampered with - and consumption thereof - I know she's going to struggle. I know her too well.

The point is that I made an effort to say "hey, if you wake up and you decide not to do it, that's cool. You can do whatever you want to, or not, it's entirely up to you, and I will support you," because I am the world's best husband and lover, the order of which switches hour-to-hour.

Anyway, we'll see how her fast goes tomorrow. I'd give it a 60 / 40 chance. Which way? I'm not sure, yet.

After I returned from *Bean There, Done That* under the blazing sun, I went to a popular game store to have a look at their summer offers. I found four Playstation 4 games for £20 (roughly $35) that I had been meaning to buy several months ago.

Oh, go on, then. Since you asked. They were: *South Park (The Fractured but Whole), Call of Duty WWII, Carmageddon*, and *Just Cause 3*.

Why am I telling you this? Well, I want to reveal my thought process today.

I dunno about you but I suffer quite badly from buyer's remorse. You know when you buy an expensive thing? You feel good about it when you hand the cash over… but seconds later you think twice and wonder if you'd made the right decision. I did the same with my extremely lean collection video games and Blu Rays. Each and every time.

Today, I saw the 4-for-£20 offer sticker and found one game, and before I knew it, I had four in my hand. I went to the counter and paid for them, returned to my apartment block, took *The Lazy Route* to the 5th floor, and downed an entire glass of water.

I didn't think twice about handing over my credit card to pay for them. The chances of me actually loading just *two* of these games onto my console are slim, let alone actually playing them. The point is that I bought them - on impulse, as ever - and felt pretty good about it.

Fast-forward to me putting Amelia to bed (bless her, her daily commute, and full day of office work) and we decide that over a period of a fortnight (or "two weeks" for those of you don't know. See? Learning all the time) we would have had take-out at least five times. All the usual suspects - famous chicken places, burger joints were in play, not to mention the occasional "midnight snack" we used to get from anywhere open 24 hours a day. Take KFC, for example. A trip there sets us back £17 for the two of us. McDonalds is about the same. Chinese takeout is more expensive for both of us, clocking in around the £26 mark. Indian? It's rare, but you can probably double the Chinese figure, especially if we sit-in at the restaurant and factor in the drinks and tip.

We figured the takeout average to set us back £20. You really don't need to be a mathematician to work out just how much money we've saved by eschewing them thus far.

In case you have dyscalculia (yes, it's a thing - Google it) here goes:

5 days x £20 = £100 ($127 *approx.*)

£20 for four video games? It's a no-brainer. Actually, what it is *is a reward*. Four pretty ornamental things to put on my already-impressive DVD shelf when we move to our new house so I can show them off to the friends I don't have and people who'll never, ever visit.

In case you're wondering, that takeout figure is about £2,700 per year, or thereabouts. It's a bit of a misnomer, really, because that implies I'll never eat takeout again - and that's just wrong. Once I hit my goal weight? I can have whatever I want, whether it's McDonald's, KFC, Burger King (we don't have Wendy's or Taco Bell in the UK. We still have to catch up with the Americans, although I'm sure it's just a matter of time) and whatever else I want. As long as it's *not too often* and I book in a bit of a *fasting* cleanse shortly thereafter.

But I keep forgetting. Once I reach my target weight of 12 stone / 167 lbs, I'll be slim. The resulting blimp my body experiences from the occasional cheeseburger will probably show less. Won't it? God, I hope so. I can't be one of those people who only has to look at a milkshake and - *BLOIK!* - my double chin bursts back out. I'm just recording my thinking in the "here and now" for posterity. From now on, as per the Roger Ebert quote that opened the introduction (don't think I've forgotten, by the way!), I intend to eat healthy and fast regularly. When I re-read that last sentence I *thought* I'd written "I intend to eat fast food and eat regularly" and nearly took it out. Please, *please* make sure you read this book twice, and double-check your notes just to be sure.

Remember to check out the essential references at the end of the book for more on this, Andrew. And if you, dear reader, want to do the same, then that's fine, too.

Okay, I've started my 48-hour fast.

I'll eat again at 8 pm Saturday night. A tin of tuna and a couple of hard boiled eggs; all protein to get my body used to food again in a *non-stupid way*.

Until then, at about 8 am tomorrow morning (twelve hours henceforth) my body will have burned most of the carbohydrates in my body and set about looking for fat to burn. According to the genius Dr. Jason Fung, the fat-burning process really kicks in on days two and three, and continues burning at basically the same rate until you stop. Friday and Saturday are fat-killer days, and the less movement I do, the more I'll burn. Go figure.

Wow, there are just *three* more entries to go - not counting Kebab Monday. So, technically-speaking that's *four*. How can I not report on Kebab Monday for all you wonderful readers?

The moment the last strand of lamb meat / French fry burrows down my throat and hits my stomach, the next fast will begin. Next week (long after these diary entries are finished), I plan to do a three or four-day fast till Thur / Fri. Let's face facts. My body will have a zillion calories and nutrients to chew through, so I'm all set. The key word is *gradual*, here. Do everything, at every stage, gradually. More importantly; know *why* you're doing it. Spend a bit of time getting to know how it works.

I'll leave this July 4 entry on a more touching (literally) note. After dinner, I sat with Amelia on the sofa and gave her a massage. We're very touchy-feeling at almost every moment we have, even over more than a decade of marriage. Any chance to touch, bite, stroke, fondle, lightly-slap, hug, or *whatever* - we do it.

She felt me back while I was attending to her feet. She's quite upset about my earlobes shrinking. Her fingers prodded around my "titch bits" - they'd shrunk, too. And my tummy. And my legs.

Her husband is disappearing before her very eyeballs! Who knows? It might have prompted the idea that came shortly after to join me in a fast. Finally, positive confirmation from the one woman who has access to my body (not that any men do, you understand). She tore the band aid off to discover the wound on my hip had reddened like an embarrassed red-headed stepchild and, much like that cruel analogy I just made, was bleeding clear liquid. My pants had rubbed against it and made it swell. It might need ice or something. I'll check back on it tomorrow.

Remember, *The Hunger Diaries* is for me, and me alone. A document of what I did and didn't do, and how I felt and how I changed and adapted. Without my recording each day in vivid detail, perhaps it would've failed? I'd recommend to anyone undertaking something profound to do the same - yeah, even *you*. Remind me to include that on the bulleted list at the end of this book.

Final thought: If my fricken *earlobes* can shift the weight, then *surely* my "titch bits" can, too?

I guess I'll find out in a few months' time. You won't, though, because this is just a two-week journal... that is, unless, you email me to ask and find out...

Day 12, or:
"Grinder (with an 'e')"

"Catch on fire and people will come from miles to see you burn."
- John Wesly

<u>Friday, July 5th, 2019</u>

I have a confession to make.

Everything I thought I knew about losing weight was *wrong*. So very, *very* wrong…

I started it all wrong.

Like an uneducated fool, I jumped head-first into a process I knew virtually nothing about, and elected to follow the Bale / Jillette *whatever-it-was* system of attempting to lose weight to discover that it wouldn't work in the long-term and probably backfire. I think back to all those contestants on *The Biggest Loser* and see they've piled the weight back on. They have the wrong idea. Watch the video I'll inevitably include at the end of the book to see why this happened. It's important.

It's not about the "eat less, move more".

It's all about the fasting.

Earlier this week I noticed real results - both physically and mentally - with regard to my 48-hour fast. When I told Amelia I was doing this she was concerned. I guess anyone would be. It seems this process of burning fat, despite scientific backing by numerous qualified individuals isn't well-known just yet.

Anyway…

Amelia did indeed do her fast today. She seemed relatively happy, and keen to know a little more about the process. She had her coffee and green tea and salt etc. It was a *punitively* hot day today. Nobody can blame her for keeping still and being cool.

Like her, I consumed the same water fasting liquids all day. I drove to *Bean There, Done That* today, although I did take *The Lazy Route* back up to the fifth floor when I returned home.

I wasn't hungry at all today. A couple of tiny *threats* of hunger were quickly allayed by a glass of filtered water. I've had two black coffees and two green teas, both with a pinch of Himalayan salt.

My mom calls me on a Friday evening around 9 pm for our weekly catch up. It usually happens around the time I'm halfway through a KFC bucket. She doesn't know about *The Hunger Diaries* but she knows I'm working on a "project." I've been maddeningly vague about it. It's okay, though; she'd rather not know and have it be a surprise. I'll surprise her, for sure. I plan to visit for a short break just as the paperback of this book comes out, so she'll get a double-whammy of *the answer* in one hit.

It was amusing to hear her ask "Oh, have you had your dinner?" to which my response was "Oh, yeah."

Technically-speaking I wasn't lying; tonight's "dinner" was a second green tea, followed by a dessert consisting of filtered water.

It's now 1:10 am on Saturday morning as I type this very sentence; twenty-seven hours since I digested those strawberries and a banana. I'm not hungry now, either.

It's possible you can tell this from my prose - I feel *great*. I'm about to enter a state know as *Ketosis*, which I won't explain here, but trust me - it's a *good* thing. My body will rest during sleep (duh!), and when I wake up, it'll be subsisting on my stored fat for energy, which means it'll burn, burn, *burn*.

Amelia will *break* her *fast* tomorrow at some point. If she goes until 8pm, then that'll be her first ever 48-hour fast. I don't know if she'll make it, but I *am* curious to see how her mood and general approach to life is affected tomorrow. I suspect it'll be positive.

This revelation I'm about to tell you fascinates me. Do you remember when Amelia revealed that certain people would never tell others about what they're doing? That they're so secretive, and consider it personal? Yeah, that. Now, it's happening with me. What Amelia doesn't know is that I don't intend to break my fast on Saturday night - rather, I'll continue it *for a week*. I want to break the news to her gently, so am drip-feeding her the information on a day-by-day basis so she doesn't stop me. And she won't stop me if, day-to-day, she sees I'm not dying. I stress that I am only *considering* fasting for an entire week. If I do, that's Kebab Monday well and truly done for. We'll see.

Funny how the world works, though, isn't it? Amelia was correct. It's true; I'm finding I'm doing a personal, *diet* version of that very same ideology. We do truly do keep our dietary endeavors secret, and that fact tells me that my decision to tell *nobody* about it was precisely the right thing to have done.

Tomorrow, no matter the weather, I *will* walk the two miles to *Bean There, Done That* and back. I'll inevitably get some sun, too, and God alone knows I need more of those kinds of vitamins. I'll walk and take *The Lazy Route* and exercise with my thigh master and hand grip as I have been doing intermittently throughout the days since I received them.

I discovered two interesting things today. The first is a small one, but the second is gigantic.

One.

We've all experienced this, but it's more acute in a heatwave and when you're guzzling water for hydration. *Dry mouth.* I was driving home (past the house we're about to move into sometime this century) and noticed my mouth was really quite dry. No water was available till I got home, and I had five flights of stairs to climb beforehand.

I found a way to lubricate my mouth naturally. You can try it right now as you hold this book in your hands, and it'll take five seconds.

Grind the side of your tongue with your teeth. Do it gently, and slowly.

Did you find an influx of saliva rush into your mouth? Cool, right?

Imagine how handy that will be when you're somewhere you can't drink. Obviously don't chew or swallow your tongue because that's just *stoopid*. Be careful. Saliva will appear, eventually.

And now, the second thing…

Remember when I told you that it would be good to "up" my calorie count in order to spin my metabolism faster? Turns out I was wrong; at least in terms of rapid weight loss, and I *hate* that phrase. *Weight loss*. I've realized I am not - and never have been - in the weight loss business. I am in the fat burning business. Why? Because if you just accept that one begets the other, then everything falls into place.

This only applies during my journey to each Goal #1. It's not what you eat, but *when*.

It's becoming clear to me that reducing my calorie intake was only *half* the battle. A bit like when Chevy Chase drove all that way to Wally World in *National Lampoon's Vacation* only to find out that it was closed. He held the manager at gunpoint and got what he wanted, but he probably wished he'd called ahead.

I'd like to remind you (Andrew) and *you* (dearest reader) that I only have one goal. Can you remember what it is? It's not to become a muscle-bound sex machine (although that sounds like a great follow-up Goal #2, I'll make a note of that) or maybe I'll do some online research when Amelia is out so I can *<Editor's Comment: No, Andrew. Just no>*.

No, my goal (as you already know) is to reach 12 stone / 167 lbs / 67 kg by my 41st birthday.

Yesterday, you'll recall me saying it had been 243 years since the American Declaration of Independence, or: A More Violent Form of Brexit, Before Brexit. *Americexit.* Well, it's exactly 94 days until my birthday at the time of writing this very sentence. That's a little over three months / twelve weeks.

Can it be done? Hmm.

I really haven't done too much today. I'm *fast*-approaching (hoho!) my twenty-fourth hour of water fasting (coffee / green tea / pinch of salt / filtered water) and I haven't been hungry at all, and it's not likely to happen, now. What have I done today? I checked out a few things and made some calculations. It was *bound* to happen sooner or later.

Before I show you my findings, I NEED TO STRESS (yes, caps!) that I suck at math, and am in no way qualified to conclude anything scientific, let alone act an authority on any of this - *just like you.*

I'm going to write my theorem in two versions; the first, for overweight / obese / curious, but thin / intrigued adults, and the second, streamlined version for two-year-old children. Here we go…

<u>VERSION ONE</u>

Fat-Burning Theory For Adults Who Suck at Math & Science but Want to *Not* be a Fat Pig, Anymore, Thank You.

Now, I've promised (Vow #4) to *not* weigh myself before Monday July 8th - and I'm sticking to it. I need data. So, I'm going to take the data on myself at the beginning of this process. The tools I'm about to use are all available to you at the end of the book, clearly labeled, and why you might want to use them (clue: you need them, so don't argue with me). It'll come as no surprise that one can find all these tools with astounding ease by just typing it into Google, which is how I found them.

Anyway, a recap…

Height: 5'11"

Weight: 217 lbs / 15.5st

Easy enough so far, right?

Okay, next up… apparently, 1 lb of body fat (in your "titch bits", belly, wherever) is equivalent to 3,500 calories. Cool, right?

All I need to know is how much fat I'm carrying in lbs on my ghastly, flabby body. So, let's go have a look, by visiting the BFC (Body fat Calculator) online which, *gasp!*, will reveal how much fat I have in my ghastly, flabby body.

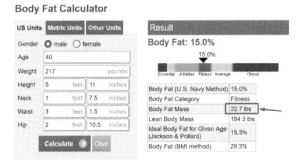

In case you cannot see the image clearly enough on your out-of-date reading device (ebook user only, you paperback guys rock - remind me to sign your copy when we meet), I typed in my age, gender (*two-spirit* was missing, wtf?), weight, height etc, and it turns out ~~I am~~ my body is:

Fat = 15% *(Really? Seems a bit low to me. I mean, it's good to know, but who cares?)*

Body Fat Mass = 32.7 lbs *(Aha! That's what I wanted. Perfect.)*

Okay, I'll pause here to let you digest (snigger!) that information while I take questions from the audience. Yes, sir, you at the back?

Anecdotally, if someone had told me thirteen days ago that I would be *lighter* right now *and* typing what I'm typing, I'd have completely written them off as insane and stuffed another double bacon cheeseburger in my mouth. Honestly, just re-reading all this ASTONISHES me. I guess it speaks to the nature of impulsiveness. Thirteen days ago I made a snap decision out of the blue to do this, and here we are. Go figure.

Anyway, let's get to the good bit.

So, here's your new, favorite author (Andrew Mackay) carrying around a combined 32.7 lbs in his "titch bits" and buttocks and belly and the padding around his *<removed>*. At least, that was the case when I started. I hope Monday's weigh-in has reduced, but I'll guess we'll find out.

According to various sources, it takes 3,500 calories to burn 1 lb of fat.

You can see where I'm going with this, can't you? And if you can't, don't worry; two weeks ago I was in your position. Let me *really* "layman" it up for y'all.

If it takes 3,500 calories to burn 1 lb of fat (and I have 32.7 of them)… I kinda need to know how long it'll take to burn.

Let's be really silly, here. Let's pretend I CAN burn 3,500 calories per day. I can't, you understand, but for the sake of argument let's assume it can be done.

It'll take 32.7 days - or 33 days if we're rounding up - to burn off all my body fat. Yeah, makes sense.

With me so far? Okay, all good.

Whoa, hold up. *32.7 lbs of fat?* That's, like, the weight of a small child. *Damn.* Hey, I tell you what, why don't we convert 32.7 lbs into calories and *really* depress myself.

(1 lb = 3,500 calories)

32.7 x 3,500 calories = 114,450 calories.

Yikes. I'm carrying 114,450 calories in my body. Ahhhh, *they need burning.*

I need to burn 114,450 calories into dust. I'll leave that to my metabolism, mostly because I have no choice in the matter.

I need to know what my **metabolism** (i.e. our general life-preserving process a.k.a. all the organs and stuff working to keep us alive a.k.a the dude inside us with the flamethrower who's burning all that fat after he's spent 12 hours burning through what I last ate) **rate** actually is. How many calories I am naturally burning off by simply being human? Please, please be 3,500 calories (lol, etc).

To find that out, I need to calculate my Basal Metabolic Rate. Yeah, I don't know what basal means, either. Like baseline? Whatever. Let's visit the BMR calculator, input my fat ass's data, and see how many calories Andrew Mackay's body likes to burn on a daily basis.

BMR Calculator

The *Basal Metabolic Rate (BMR) Calculator* estimates your basal metabolic rate—the amount of energy expended while at rest in a neutrally temperate environment, and in a post-absorptive state (meaning that the digestive system is inactive, which requires about 12 hours of fasting).

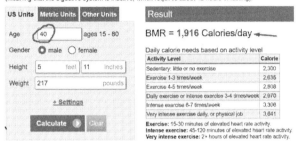

Activity Level	Calorie
Sedentary: little or no exercise	2,300
Exercise 1-3 times/week	2,635
Exercise 4-5 times/week	2,808
Daily exercise or intense exercise 3-4 times/week	2,970
Intense exercise 6-7 times/week	3,306
Very intense exercise daily, or physical job	3,641

Exercise: 15-30 minutes of elevated heart rate activity.
Intense exercise: 45-120 minutes of elevated heart rate activity.
Very intense exercise: 2+ hours of elevated heart rate activity.

That's interesting.

At my height and weight, I burn approximately 1,916 calories a day *by just being me*. The calculator reaches this conclusion by factoring in my activity level. If you're sedentary (as authors mostly are, sitting around all day and don't move much) then I actually chew through 2,300 calories per day. The extreme end of that spectrum (very intense exercise daily, or physical job), tells me I'd be burning 3,641 calories. I've been walking quite a bit and exercising lightly for a few days now that I have the equipment, not to mention taking *The Lazy Route* at least once per day.

Hmmm. So what you're telling me is that *if I exercise more*, I'll have a higher metabolic rate to spend burning? That if, say, 500 calories of my day is food, and I exercise like a banshee to clock in that 3,641 calorie number above, my metabolism will burn through those first 500 first and then find the remaining 3,141 in my fat stores? Per day? Seeing that 3,500 calories equals one pound of fat?

Okay, you've got my attention, now. Tell me more...

My back-of-the-cigarette-packet calculations says I burn around 2,500 calories per day. Roughly. I mean, there are fluctuations and other things to consider that are far too complex for me to really understand, so I'm not even going to attempt to write about them here. What matters is that I am *me*, sedentary, *and* getting a modest amount of not-especially-taxing physical exercise. About the same amount of exercise as a recently-dumped teenage girl who can't get off Instagram on her cell phone whilst walking 3 km to McDonald's to get three milkshakes.

Being something of a sadist, I enjoy the 1,916 calories result. To make life easier, let's round that result to 2,000 if, for no other reason, than to satisfy my obsessive compulsive disorder which, as it happens, keeps my expectations really low. My body spends 2,000 calories per day burning, uh… oh, I seemed to have finished my sentence.

All I need to decide now is *what* my metabolism is going to burn. In an ideal world, it'd be incinerating years-old fat currently propping up my belly, and consigned it to the dustbin of ex-obese Andrew, and have it stay there for the rest of recorded time. Yeah, I think that one *truly* tops the list of my priorities.

Incidentally, before we look at this last part (deciding how my body will kill fat), my spectacles are *once again* falling down my face in quite an annoying way. The goddess optician girl only tightened them yesterday. *And my spectacles, too.* I'm not sweating and my skin isn't oily, or anything, I swear. This is ridiculous. I keep on having to stop typing and push them up. I'll have the girl tighten them tomorrow (the spectacles, not that other thing you just thought of. Oh. You *weren't* thinking that? Well, you are now. You're welcome).

Okay, I've got you back in the game with that carefully constructed joke, just there. Welcome back.

I have 2,000 calories per day to spend burning. Potentially more, if I exercise like a demon. It can be burning *fat*, or food I just ate.

So, how much food should I consume on a daily basis?

If I "take in" 1,000 calories of food, my metabolism will demolish those first, and then move onto a further 1,000 burning fat.

Or, if I "take in" 500 calories, it'll use the remaining 1,500 calories to burn fat.

Hang on a moment. What if... I "take in" zero calories (prolonged fasting)? Yeah. 2,000 calories. We'll call it three-quarters of a pound, or 0.75 lbs.

That's the "idiot's guide" to how this all works. I know this is true because I am a *genuine* idiot. Of course, it doesn't *quite* work like this, but it's as damn near close as I'm satisfied with.

The key is to reduce your calorie intake and maximize the calorie... uh, *outtake*? Or whatever it's called when calories exit the body.

Using this extremely stupid, ill-advised and inaccurate method of calculating how to lose fat, I'll utilize my patented **Fool Yourself** method to conclude that:

In order to burn 114,450 calories at optimum metabolic "incineration" rate will take **57.8 (58) days** of continuous, prolonged water fasting to reach my target weight of 12 stone / 167 lbs / 67 kg

I'm not prepared to do a 58-day water fast, although people do it. The record is 328 days but now we're getting into fatally-obese territory. The guy who did it was something like 6,000,000,000 lbs and dropped to around 160 lbs in just over a year. I'm fat but I'm not *that* fat, thanks. My body needs protein and "good" fats every so often. Besides, I don't want to end up with *no* body fat whatsoever. I mean that's just silly. A healthy body fat percentage would be around 14-24%, depending on your daily level of activity.

I'm now twelve days into the process, and I'm probably lighter than my initial readings *and* I don't want to burn it all. This tells me I have a fighting chance of hitting my goal weight by my desired deadline. With that, here's my final, final, *final* conclusion.

I'll continue to do my 22:2 (22 hours fasting, 2 hours feeding) on the days I eat. I'll get a good ten hours of my metabolism burning fat each day. I will alternate this with prolonged (3-5 continuous days) water fasts. The fat burning process really kicks in on day two, and goes gangbusters on days 3 and 4, although on day 4, you do start to feel a bit weak, so I hear.

Remember how I said I was going to do a 48-hour fast and eat again Saturday night? Yeah. That just changed. I've lengthened the period, and moved it back to Sunday night at least. A 72-hour fast. I'm still mulling-over a week-long fast and very 50/50 on it.

If these calculations are correct (and believe me, they're probably not), I expect to shed around *one whole pound* by then. I'll introduce my body to lean protein just before bed on Sunday - just before I get tired and hungry *because* I ate - in order to prep my body for *Kebab Monday*. I don't want to *shock* myself thin, or antagonize my body by eating nothing for three days and suddenly ramming a sweaty lamb kebab and fries down my throat.

I need to think ahead to the long-term, though; keep the weight off once I nail my target figure. I figure 1,000 calories, or thereabouts, on the days I do eat right now is realistic. As I approach my goal weight around September (ish) and can see the results, I'll gently apply the brakes and "up" my calorie intake in increments towards 2,000 calories per day. *Gradually*. Why? So when I hit my goal weight, I'll return to "normal" on a "normal" 2,000 calories eating "normal" food that's good and healthy. Of course, I expect that last stretch to the finish line to drag on a few days more because my food / burn ratio will have closed. Also, psychologically, it'll help. The data suggest it will work, so it's worth a shot.

<u>VERSION TWO</u>
Fat-Burning Theory For Two-Year-Old Children.

Once upon a time there was a really fat man who had a big tummy and stupid, bouncy breasts. So he ate no food and did walks and climbed stairs till all the wobbly bits went away. When the fat man got hungry he drunked water lots and lots to make the hungry go away. Sometimes he drank yucky black coffee with all salt that adults drank because he was really sad. So the fat man stopped eating bad food, like Mr. Cheeseburger who wanted to give him a heart attack, and Mr. Soda who was nice but really bad inside because he was secretly hiding a white powder that could kill him. But the fat man didn't die because all the food he ate months and years ago was still inside of him and that's what made his belly and boobies really big like a lady's so he stopped eating food while his body got rid of all the fat with a big sword and then he was thin again and he was really happy because he didn't need his mobility scooter to go to Walmart any more.

Day 13, or:
"Hall of Mirrors"

"Once you have dialog starting,
you know you can break down prejudice."
- Harvey Milk

<u>Saturday, July 6th, 2019</u>

RI-II-II-IIP-P!

Off came the the band aid, and - shock, horror! - my fricken hip wound has gotten *worse*. The look on Amelia's face was a picture of horror and told me everything I seriously hoped what I knew.

"Jeez. It's gone all raw-red and inflamed."

"What?" I asked, worried.

I wondered what that stinging sensation was when I was walking around, but I can't go walking *without* my pants; without underwear, possibly, but then my fabulously well-endowed appendage would get some pants-rub action, too, and tent me for most of the day, which will slow down my walk. *Something of a Snatch-22, if you will.* Besides, the very *last* thing I need as I accompany Amelia

213

to *Shoes* is for those women in the make-up department seeing me walk around with a concealed erection (the size of two tins of Red Bull on top of each other) and having me fast-tracked onto the sex offender's register before we've even reached the *Maybelline* counter.

"Seriously," Amelia said, having not heard that last paragraph because I've only just typed it, "You need to get down to the doctor's and have that looked at. It looks bad. It looks sore."

"It *is* sore," I huffed as I made the mistake of pressing my fingers around the outer inflamed bit. "Ouch. I just knew my pants were rubbing against it and making it worse."

Amelia rose to her feet and closed the conversation with a look on her face that suggested I shouldn't dare argue with the next sentence that came out of her mouth, which was, "Go visit the doctor first thing Monday. You have more chance of being seen if you just turn up."

"Yes, okay. Good idea."

I pulled up my pants, and recounted the events of the day…

I figured out why I was salivating so much during the first few days. It's because I was eating generally good food (tuna, apples, bananas etc) for lunch, and then waiting around six hours for dinner. Then, I had another eight hours to go till I went to bed.

Those hours of not eating (apart from the morning because *breakfast*, obviously) were the worst. I salivated *a lot* and kept spitting everywhere like a cowboy chewing a fistful of tobacco in some tenth-rate western. It wasn't until last weekend that I discovered why I was salivating like a bulldog at a peanut butter carnival. It certainly wasn't until I started fasting that I proved the theory once and for all.

I'm writing this sentence at 1 am in the morning of Sunday, July 7th. Technically, tomorrow is the now-famous *Kebab Monday*. It's been 53 hours since food last past my lips, not that my mind or stomach knows it. I'm not hungry and, apart from the occasional twinge of hunger (sated by a glass of water), I've gotten quite used to *not eating at all*.

Now, I know what you're thinking - holy… *moly*, Andrew, you nut case! What on Earth do you think you're doing?

Funny you should ask that. It's not *what* I'm doing but *what's* happening. What I *think* I'm doing is allowing three important things to occur. It's all based on scientific studies *and* being demonstrated right this very second by me - the ultimate test subject.

1: I think my body is burning through my stored fat. All my flabby parts are tightening quite dramatically. I'm constantly having to pull up my size 40" trousers. They've begun to slip due to movement and rub against the left hip, causing me some insane irritation. My glasses continue to slip down my face despite my not sweating or skin getting all oily. The fact that my *head* is shrinking is some Jivaroan tribe witchcraft nonsense, right there.

2: If #1 is true then this *must* mean that **my insulin is way, way down** - low enough to allow the decades-of-stored fat-burning process to occur. Don't take my word for it - check out all the reference links at the end of the book backing this evidence up scientifically. My blood sugar must be down, too. I'm not cold and *hangry* like I was when I was enacting the *eat less, move more* method for the first six days of this adventure.

3: I think I'm **more active and more alert**. I'm sleeping better, too. I'm out-for-the-count the second my head hits the pillow. I wake up full of the joys of Spring and not hungry.

Speaking of being active, I walked the two miles to *Bean There, Done That* today. It was a bright and sunny day but it didn't matter. I figured what the heck? Get my sweat on. I didn't sweat at all, in fact.

A curious happened when I was walking. I noticed my energy levels enacting their bragging rights and making me move quicker. If you're fat like I *still* am (sadly, this is a long process, which is why Ebert's opening quote is ultra-important), then you'll know you spend a lot of your time hunched over slightly in order to minimize your gut and hanging breasts. You're fooling nobody, my friend, by doing that. Years of doing this means your body will evolve into a fricken question mark when viewed in profile by others.

My head was up, my chest pushed out, and I had an ultra-confident stride - no doubt aided by opting to take *The Lazy Route* over the past few days. It all helped. The walk was really, really enjoyable. I can't wait to do it again. A four-mile round trip, and most of it in the sun… I mean, the closest I can describe the feeling was one of semi-euphoria; feeling lighter and having a bit of a bounce in your step.

I reached *Bean There, Done That* to see Unlucky Number 8 taking up most of the right-hand side of the storefront, sitting there and chatting to someone on her phone. She caught me glancing at her. We made eye contact the briefest of moments. I quickly averted my gaze to the door as I pushed it open only to see her smiling in my peripheral vision.

What happened next will astound you, as it did me… so I'm saving it for the *end* of this chapter.

A little later in the afternoon I made a discovery that I think you'll find interesting.

Amelia wanted to go to *Shoes* to buy… girlie *stuff*. I dunno, lipstick and blusher and all that looks the same to me. Thank God my interest in cross-dressing is limited because, knowing me, I'd end up going outside with concealer on my lips.

As is typical when a guy attends a cosmetics place with their significant other, they tend to stand around, bored out of their mind, trying to *not* look like a dribbling pervert. There are scant few areas to look at while this happens to your average, "spoken-for" guy. I don't mind, though, as it gives me a chance to daydream my next book, or the next chapter of whatever I'm writing.

Standing by the rows of lipsticks, I decided to look UP. Guess what I found? My own face staring back at me from above. About a foot or so above my head was a tilted mirror angling down at my face. Of course, this is designed for women to apply some sample lipstick and see how it looks on them.

But something didn't sit *quite* right.

Then, I noticed I didn't have a double chin - and the reason for that was because I had to tilt my head up to see my face. A textbook way to rid yourself of your double-chin. Now, us fatties know *damn well* that when we visit the bathroom and accidentally catch our own reflection we tend to stick our heads out a bit to reduce the ghastly flab under our chins. Guess what that act is called? Yeah, **Fool Yourself** - *and certainly nobody else.*

Then, my three years of training for my media and film degree at the taxpayer's expense (thanks, Tony Blair!) came flooding back. One of the modules we undertook was on advertising. For example, did you know that major clothing stores have fitting rooms with large mirrors installed in them? Fair enough, it's what we expect; but a practice goes on that's not unlike those Hall of Mirrors at the carnival - you know the ones; they're all bendy and stuff and you look stupid and it's funny.

What if… those large mirrors in the fitting rooms were curved *eeeevvvveeerrr-so-slightly*? To the point that you can't see it with the naked eye. We're talking fractions of a centimeter. Or millimeters, if you want to get all pedantic about it.

The result? A slimmer *you*. Of course, these mirrors don't resemble those obsolete curved TV screens as that'd be too obvious. The resultant effect, though, is not unlike a propulsive encouragement for the ***Fool Yourself*** methodology buried deep within your decision-making. A thinner *you*. In my mind it plays out a bit like this.

[Enter stage right: Overweight woman enters the fitting room and puts on the dress]

"Ugh, I don't want to look at that mirror. Okay, I guess I'll have to so I can see how this dress look—... *OH!* Hang on. Wow, look at me. I'm not the hideous and overweight rhinoceros I thought I was! Daaayaaam, I look pretty damn *fine* in this dress. Wow. *Etc.*"

[Woman buys dress without hesitation. She gets home, wears it again, sees she's fat after all, and returns it the next day for a refund - but not before having a good cry on the phone to her mother for two hours and the world explodes in a nuclear holocaust.]

You might have already known the *Hall of Mirrors* effect was happening. So, treat it as a reminder that it continues to go on. If you *didn't* know this before you read it just now, may I ask you a question?

Thanks.

How do you feel about things, now?

It turns out that, not only are we wonderfully skilled in the magic of **Fool Yourself** *(dammit, I NEED to patent this - and fast)*, but large companies *(CoughDietSodaCough)* use carefully calibrated techniques to aid the methodology, too. How long has this been going on for? Go on, have a guess.

Answer: Since at least the 1950s.

Back then, we didn't have McDonald's, KFC, Wendy's, Arby's, Taco Bell, Pizza Hut, etc, on the industrial scale we have today, despite many of them starting life in the 1950s. Back then, and up until around the late eighties, meals were largely a home-cooked affair. The fast food places were a treat, and infrequent. Their portions were smaller, too. We didn't have Costco, which meant we weren't buying Hershey bars by the planet-load. Thus, we didn't have a cupboard full of dangerously sugary snacks to gorge on every ten minutes before the next meal. The temptation simply didn't exist. We binge-eat in exactly the same way we binge-watch, now. *Binge* - the byword of modern times. Much like the yet-to-be-invented Netflix, we couldn't "eat on demand" and "binge eat" our favorite TV shows when it suited us. We had to race home in time to catch the latest episode of *Full House* / have our family dinner in the evening. Missed it? Tough. There was no Tivo. No VCRs. Our laziness had consequences.

Refrigerators were smaller back then, too. Freezers were a luxury, which meant that if we couldn't afford one, there was no ice cream and perishable foods that'd last longer than a week, thus, fewer clogged arteries to deliver our myocardial infarctions years later. We hadn't heard of dieting because, frankly, it didn't exist. Society was not overweight. Well, I say "we" - back in the fifties, the world would be experiencing a cruel deprivation of its greatest, living, Pulitzer-prize-deserving author Andrew Mackay for *at least* another twenty years. (1978, in case you can't count backwards from 40).

Think about the last commercial (radio, TV, whatever) you saw. Was it for fruit? How about kale and spinach? Of course it wasn't. Let's not over-egg the pudding (lol, obviously), here. I'm not talking about the food, rather *the offer*. It's not the food that is compelling us. We've already got the food figured out. It's the *idea* of *value* + FOMO (Fear of Missing Out) we fall for…

ONE: *"Buy One Get SEVENTEEN Free on chocolate bars!"*

[Save money. Get fat.]

TWO: *"It's Monday, and you're stuck with the same old, boring lunch. But not today. Us cool kids here at <insert company name> enjoy our Mondays with the all-new, limited edition barbecue chicken-flavor wrap with garlic mayonnaise until 3 pm. Only $1.99"*

[Mouth-watering temptation timed for 11 am in the morning, underpinned with a subtle sound effect of sizzling meat. I work, too, what a coincidence! And I eat lunch. God, I'm hungry. Monday? Ugh, beginning of a five-day working week. I deserve a treat. 3 pm you say? I'd better get down there. Human beings are hardwired to never miss a deal. $1.99? Ah, screw it, I'll have *four*, please. [Oh, and add a large order of fries and soda to go with it.]

THREE: *"Your family will go nuts for our new STENT CRISPIES; fortified with all your daily vitamins and NO added sugar! Our cute little mascots, Snack, Crackle, and Flop love it, too! It's the best-selling, wholesome brand our customers have loved since 1928. You and your families' arteries can't help but widen for STENT CRISPIES's tasty and natural goodness."*

[Yeah, and what about the sugar content? Oh, no *added* sugar? *Added*. Okay, I'll give you a bowl of table sugar, then. It's okay, though. I didn't *add* any sugar to it.]

All of this is either going to sound a) familiar to you, or b) like a messed-up conspiracy theory.

If you fall into the first category (as I suspect you do) then well done. You can keep reading.

If you fall into the latter category then you're astoundingly stupid with precisely *zero* social wherewithal and common sense that I DEMAND you stop reading and ask for a refund.

Better still, go and tell all your equally-dumb little chums that you hated this book *and* then leave a one-star review at Amazon. They say there's no better form of advertising than word of mouth. A one-star review from an illiterate moron is worth approximately 500 five-star reviews from a *normal* person. Why? Because intelligent people *laugh* at your badly spell checked reviews that say: *"Andew is meen and I didn't loose weyt and he said bad things and he neds a proof radar,"* and make me seem like a decent dude whose book is worth buying.

Now go away - *and stay fat and stupid.*

[Andrew goes outside for a smoke to calm down.]

[Oh, crap. He's coming back… quick, look busy…]

Hey guys. Look, I'm sorry you had to read that last bit. I needed to do a bit of house cleaning before the end of the book. I can't have some a-hole who can only count to eleven with his zipper undone going on to try what I'm doing, only to kill themselves because they've confused inches for feet, or pounds for kilograms ala Nigel Tufnel in *This is Spinal Tap*. (*"Stone'endge"*) Honestly, I question the intelligence level of people, sometimes.

Oh, speaking of questions…

One question I'm getting asked over and over again by absolutely nobody because they don't know I'm doing this is:

What happened to the yogurt, bananas, and apples, Andrew? You lied to us. You put it on the front cover—

—Wait, wait, *stop*. I get it. Let me answer. I could point you in the direction of the above three examples, but they don't count because apples and bananas don't get much radio play.

Simply put? I didn't need them *and* they're high in sugar and fructose; the two archenemies of fat-burning process. So, you know, that's why I gave them up. Especially the low-fat yogurt because "*no added sugar.*" (Go back and read example three again if you're confused.)

Fast forward to 11 pm today. I find myself sitting in a movie theater watching Luc Bessons' latest movie, *Anna*.

Yeah, it's pretty good, since you're asking. Anyway, around thirty minutes before the film finished, I shifted my not-inconsiderable weight onto my left buttock to let out *what I thought was a little fart.*

You don't need me to tell you what happened next - but I'm going to.

An avalanche of what felt like scorching-hot molten lava streaked up inside my buttocks, forcing me to clench them together to save my underwear from drowning a messy, bowel-based death. Any sane person might have got up and left, but I figured it would be best to remain seated. You know, like when you're on a long haul flight and grind your buttocks right into the seat to create a vacuum so that when you fart the entire bubble of gas is trapped between your ass cheeks for the duration of the flight? By the time you arrive at Botswana International Airport and stand up, a five-hour-old, pungent aroma wafts through the economy cabin as everyone's trying to be the first to get their luggage out of the overhead coffins.

This little interlude is brought to you by Too Much Information; for all your undesired knowledge needs.

The film ended and I completely forgot about the incident. It seemed that my underwear had, indeed, caught a glimpse of what I *hadn't* been eating. So, very carefully, I walked like the Duracell Bunny in *ultra-sloooow-motion* to the movie theater's bathroom.

In the stall (or cubicle, if you're in the UK) I pulled everything down, took as close a peek as I could manage, and blew a sigh of relief. The damage wasn't as bad as it had *felt*. Much like the prospect of fasting, now that I think about it. Anyway, there were a few drops of ass-water, but little else. All it took was a good scrub between the cheeks to the solve the issue and allow me on my merry way back to my car.

Of course, when I got home I changed my underwear and attended to myself with a few baby wipes about an hour ago before I started writing.

The point I'm trying to make is this - when you've not eaten for fifty hours, any semblance of food clearly turns to water and will shotgun through your ring-piece and into your pants acting as a hammock. Thus, if you fast for a prolonged period of time, be *really careful*. I'm fortunate that it's only happened twice - once at home (phew!) and once at a place where a bathroom was nearby.

The second question that people who don't know about this journey just won't shut the hell up about today is… *what happened to Amelia with her fast?*

She made it to 5 pm - forty-five hours of fasting. Not a bad attempt considering it was her first time, had no preparation, and ate a lot of bad food the day (and weeks and months and years) before she began. She got through the period really well, and I'm proud of her for doing it. The benefits of her attempt probably aren't as significant as mine, but it was the mental challenge of her seeing it through that pleased me the most. She broke her fast with slices of an apple at 5 pm, then a couple of eggs at around 8 pm, followed by a small selection of the food she really likes - and crashed the hell out at about the time I left to go to the movies.

I came home around midnight, took care of my crapped-pants-extravaganza, and dumped them in the laundry. I would've confessed about my incident right there and then, but she was fast asleep in bed at the time. In fact, I've still not told her. She'll find out when she reads this paragraph. (*Soooooooorriiiiee.*)

Now, let's rewind to earlier this afternoon…

After my time at *Bean There, Done That*, I went to the opticians to get my glasses tightened because they were slipping off my face. Not to spoil what happened, but they're slipping *again* as I write this sentence. I'm not sweating and my skin hasn't any moisture.

The pretty optician girl I saw the other day was there and she recognized me immediately. She was quite surprised that they were slipping so soon after she gripped it in her fist and gave it a *damn good tug*. <Note: Insert crass innuendo here.> They have this spinning machine that does some tightening wizardry I seriously can't be bothered to comprehend, but she put my spectacles in the machine thing anyway and gave them a *bloody good seeing-to*.

I asked her if she could measure how tight she was making them, like, by millimeters or whatever, so I could put the answer in this book. But it turns out these scientists and geniuses don't actually measure how tight they make them; they go by data that any authority on the subject would use - *how it looks and feels on the patient*.

Thank heavens *real* doctors don't do this…

"Okay, Mr. Trump. Just take ten of these pills every day for two weeks and it'll clear those crabs up a treat."

"But… doctor?"

"What?"

"These are *TicTacs*."

"Shut up."

Etc.

I slipped my spectacles back on, clocked the optician girl in all her beauty, and decided ~~she~~ they ~~wasn't~~ weren't *quite* tight enough. She chuckled to herself and gave them a damn good wringing again in her hands, and then with her machine, and slid them back on my face. Prodding her immaculate fingers around my ears and forehead, and spending an inordinately long time staring at my eyes and face, she suggested I should try them out for 48 hours (because like every service in the UK - from ballet dancing to prostitution - they don't work on a Sunday) and come back and tell her she's pretty. Did I say pretty? I meant *how I was getting on with my freshly-tightened spectacles.*

Not seven bloody hours later I'm sitting in the movie theater with my right elbow perched on the armrest in order to rest my index finger on the bridge of my glasses so they don't slide down the bridge of my nose. *And my head is tilted up at the screen!*

Ugh. My head is definitely shrinking. Or the side of my face. Or my nose. Or my ears. I dunno, I give up. They're sliding *again* as I type this sentence. I hope this doesn't happen with contact lenses or laser eye surgery, else you won't be reading many new masterworks from me any time soon.

And now, we end this chapter on what happened about an hour before the pretty optician girl failed to do what I needed done the second time of asking…

[*The Hunger Diaries* returns after these messages.]

Cue dramatic music.

"Hey, you!"

"Who me?"

"Yes, you, you overweight bucket of pigeon droppings. Wanna lose weight?"

"Sure."

"But every time you try it fails and you pile the pounds back on?"

"Uh, sure. Wow, how do you know me so well?"

"Haha. Well, if you tried everything else, then you need to try the all-new *Fasting*!"

"Wow. Fasting?"

"Sure, fella. It's proven to work by medical scientists! It's easy to do and saves time because you're not buying / preparing / eating food and clearing up after, it reduces obesity and diabetes, eliminates all your blood pressure meds, regenerates cells for slower aging, *and* it's free!"

"Wow! It's free?"

"Uh-huh. *Free*. Absolutely *no money* involved. You gain time *and* lose weight!"

"Wow, cool. I'll take two bottles, please."

"Oh. Um. Bottles? No, I—"

"—No bottles? Well, how do I get this *Fasting* you speak of?"

"You, uh, just… do it."

"Oh cool. See ya."

Cut to: Fasting Inc., boardroom.

"Damnit, Karen. Our marketing for *Fasting* hasn't worked. Why is this?"

"Well, uh, sir?"

"What is it, Karen? You damn fool? Get me another line of coke and explain yourself."

"It's just that our profit margin is… zero. We've made no money from—"

"—*ZERO*?! Whaddya mean it's zero? What do I pay you for, Karen? All our other weight-loss programs are keeping me in hookers and yachts, and that's not to mention all the Big Pharma contracts we have to peddle unnecessary medications to keep people sick and we can make lots of money*."

"Sorry, sir. I guess we'll have to cease advertising *Fasting* until we can figure out how to monetize it."

"You're damn right about that."

Don't delay - start today!
Consult your doctor right now and see if Fasting is right for you and your family.

*Of course this isn't true. I'm joking.

[And now, we return to our feature presentation.]

1:30 pm. About three minutes ago I accidentally caught Unlucky Number 8's eye as I walked into *Bean There, Done That*.

Not two minutes later I took my seat at the adjoining table; maybe three feet away from her arms. I had my earphones in, listening to some talk radio dude waffle on about something or other. Occasionally, Unlucky Number 8 would look up at me and then back at her phone like a typical post-millennial.

A couple minutes later I got fed up with what I was listening to and removed my earphones and enjoyed the general ambiance.

I accidentally catch her eye again and she smiles. Of course what you're about to read is an approximation but it went something like this:

"Hey," she said from out of nowhere.

"Hey," I returned politely with an air of well-that's-the-end-of-the-conversation, then.

Next up, something weird happened that took *even me* by surprise…

"What you up to?" I asked, quite without my permission.

"Nothing," she revealed. "Just kinda sitting here. My Dad's in hospital."

Curious, I fished a bit more with an open question like an idiot, "I'm sorry to hear that. I hope he's okay?"

Then, she burst into tears. There's not much you can do in that position, is there? Very awkward if nothing else. She recovered from her initial waterworks and sniffed the grief of whatever-it-was away and let out a chuckle.

"Nah, it's okay. He'll be fine "

I needed to change the subject if for no other reason than to take her mind away from the upset.

"I have to ask you something," I chanced.

"Yeah?"

"I see you're here all the time. Do you work?"

"Nope. I had a job but they fired me."

"Oh," I said with a sneeze of sympathy.

"Yeah, and finding a new job is boring."

"Yeah, tell me about it."

"Why, what do you do?" she asked.

I was about to give her my usual "Oh, I'm an author" line but, just as that bad idea whipped from my brain to my mouth I stopped it from escaping my lips. I can't tell her I'm an author. This book will inevitably come up in conversation. There's a risk she might hunt down my work (not that teenagers read these days) and recognize "*Bean There, Done That*" and read about a grossly obese girl named "Unlucky Number 8" who's always here, and then put two and two together.

From a legal standpoint, who cares, right? I've gone to great lengths to protect her anonymity. You wouldn't be able to find this place I speak of unless I tell you personally where it is. If you go on the hunt using the information you've gleaned through the book you're going to be disappointed. Besides, knowing your luck, you'll find it and happen upon the one thirty-minute stretch she isn't there. Worse, you might mistake this girl for the wrong person and then all hell would break loose.

From a moral standpoint... ah, screw it. See the above paragraph. I can do what I like. Nobody knows any better. You don't know where this place is and (let's face facts) even if you *did*, you'd never actually go there to see what's up.

It turns out Unlucky Number 8's *real* name is "Shelley" (not her real name) - named after the actress Shelley Duvall who played Jack Nicholson's wife in *The Shining* because I adore that film and because it's much easier to do a find-and-replace in my word processor on the word "Shelley" if I decide to change it again by the time this book is published. Also, Duvall in *The Shining* and "Shelley"'s physical frame couldn't be further apart, so it's ironic, too - which, as an author, is extremely helpful.

"I, uh…" I scrambled for a career that would bore her to tears and kill the conversation dead. Thus, my brain figured out the answer quicker than it took to type this sentence. "I'm a teacher."

"Are you actually?"

"Yeah. Unfortunately."

"How come you're mostly here during lunchtime, though?"

"I teach night classes," I lied.

I *did* teach evening classes at a college years ago so I wasn't *technically* lying.

To my surprise, my desperately dull answer worked a treat and shifted the ball into her court. Shelley went on to reveal things about her. She lost her mother five years ago for a reason I don't really remember. Now - with her dad laid up in hospital - she's a bundle of nerves and can't sleep. Although she doesn't spit it out explicitly, it seems that *Bean There, Done That* acts as a sanctuary away from life, and not as a hideout to escape from the clutches of her demanding father hassling her to get a job.

I catch a quick peek under the table to see she's using an additional plastic chair to rest her right leg on. Now that my proximity to her is closer than I'm used to, I can hear her breathing; a sort of underwater snorkeling sound through her nose as if she has gills tucked behind one of those chins of hers. It sounds like when you suck the last puddle of milkshake out of the carton with a straw.

Believe me, it takes every single patient atom in my body to refrain from *what I wanted to say next* but, because I'm a coward (i.e. "know better"), I don't say it.

Here's what I *really* wanted to say.

"You know, it's not too late to fix your weight. You may feel better. It may give you more energy. It could help with landing that job you want."

In my mind, I'd suspect she'd go on to ask: "Oh, yeah? And how do you know that?"

But I don't say my first line.

Who am I to bring the subject of her weight up, anyway? She's hardly going to be the first to mention it, either.

And so both of us sit and finish our drinks *failing* to bring up the topic. Just like you and your friends do. The subject never comes up because you're too afraid to hear the truth, and your friends are too afraid of upsetting you.

I'll stride off into the blistering hot sun a few pounds lighter than I did a few days ago with a goal to reach my target weight. And Shelley? She'll waddle off in the other direction, headed inexorably towards complications in later life if she doesn't address her weight.

She's still so damn young, so there's *definitely* hope for her, yet. Without my snap decision on Saturday, June 22nd to lose weight, this diary wouldn't have happened. Without this diary my short conversation with Shelley would have stopped at "hey" and a polite smile. In other words, "Shelley" would always have been known in my mind as Unlucky Number 8; the obese and idle blob of fat cells who thinks the world owes her everything on a plate - with three side orders of deep-fried onion rings smothered in full-fat mayo.

I'm sure I don't need to spell out just how significantly my preconceived prejudices and general approach to others has changed since I started this journey.

Do I?

Fun Fact: This chapter took ninety minutes to write with a three-minute cigarette break at the 54th-hour of fasting.

Day 14, or:
"XL"

"You're fat, and look as though you should be, but you're not."
- Soap, *Lock Stock & Two Smoking Barrels (1998)*

<u>Sunday, July 7th, 2019</u>

I'm writing this sentence at 1 am on Sunday morning. It's been 77 hours since I last ate.

I slept like a baby, and have done each night I've fasted. I'm not kidding when I say I pass out the second my head hits the pillow. We all know that our cell phones can cause eye damage when we read in bed. I usually check news stories until I get tired. Now, I don't even bother looking at my phone. When I wake up I feel great. Like most mornings when I wasn't fasting I'm not hungry.

Breakfast really is the easiest meal of the day to skip. We've been told all our lives that it's the most important meal of the day. Not when you're trying to burn fat, it isn't.

After my morning coffee and advert-checking I'm keen to walk to *Bean There, Done That* but, now that it's the third day of my fast, I'm a little concerned that something

237

might happen. I'd heard that I might feel weak on the third or fourth day. Besides, Amelia wanted to go to the supermarket nearby, so we ended up driving there.

Amelia's not terribly fond of sitting outside this particular *Bean There, Done That* with me. It's on the crowded-side, especially at the weekends. Nevertheless, we sit outside and chat about the week ahead.

In the supermarket, she and I are searching for different things. I'm not even sure what she was after - presumably some items for her dinner. I'm not eating right now and it's not gone unnoticed by either of us that our grocery bill is half the amount it usually is.

I got the Tumeric powder I was looking for. Apparently it's great for separating brown and white fat which enables a faster burn. Also, apple cider vinegar. One of the links I'll provide in the outtroduction will tell you why apple cider vinegar is a necessity just before a workout. It burns a lot of fat for you, too.

I try the mixture when I get home. A drop of water, apple cider vinegar, Tumeric, and Pink Himalayan salt.

It's absolutely vile.

I've decided to name this gut-punch of a cocktail *The Wanker.*

Amelia and I venture into the shopping mall shortly after that. We're headed for the usual places when I get an idea to visit my favorite clothing store - which I'll call "S&M" - to try on some new shirts. Look, I'm no idiot. I have a ways to go until I hit my target weight, presumably around September or October, but I wanted to see what was doing with the sizes of shirt I wear.

I currently don an "XL" size, like most large men do.

We find the over-shirts and I make a beeline for the "L" shirts - in other words "Large." I slip the first one on and show Amelia, who said it looked just fine on me. The beautiful thing was that it was actually *somewhat* baggy. I'll be weighing myself for the first time tomorrow, but subtle hints about how much weight I might have lost keep rearing their heads. The shirt, the fact that my face has shrunk (hence the issue with my glasses), the car / toilet seat setting bigger, and so on. We don't purchase any of the shirts because if I do reach my goal weight of 12 stone, even a large size may be too big for me. Oh, to fit into a medium… now that *would* be something.

I start to get hungry around the time Amelia settles down for dinner. It's not important *what* she's eating, but the smell. Every night she's been eating dinner within punching distance. All of it smelled absolutely wonderful. As you already know, I love a challenge, and this is no different. Some poor guy who's fasting and not eating is in receipt of so many culinary stenches it's borderline mouth-watering - yet, it only strengthens my resolve and my determination to see this through. Whilst mouth-watering, the smell never makes me hungry. And don't get me wrong - I had my "dinner", too. A glass of water. (lol!)

I've decided not to drink coffee and / or green tea after around 6 pm as I don't want the caffeine keeping me awake for too long. So, quite literally, I'm only on filtered water for the last eight hours I'm awake.

Until today, that is.

I need to get up early to see if I can snatch a last-minute doctor's appointment first thing in the morning. They open at 8 am, and I need to get up at least an hour beforehand to make sure my guts are satisfied before I leave our apartment. My hip feels like it's red raw and it's itchy as all hell. My pants leg keeps rubbing against it and it's *definitely* not helping matters.

After my "dinner" I take a shower and dread, to a certain extent, what I'm going to see if I look down.

I peel off the plaster…

Ugh. Sure enough, the swelling has blossomed. A patch of black, wet skin, surrounded by an inflamed red stuffed-crust of a swell. It's sore to the touch. It seems to be *pulsating*. I can barely place my palm gently onto it to feel a nasty lump bubbling up underneath.

So, naturally, I shower *very* carefully. I try to avert the spray anywhere but my hip, and am ultra cautious when the inevitable soaping process rolls around.

As I lather my body, I notice my legs are damn-near svelte. It's almost as if I have no fat on them. All those times I took *The Lazy Route*, and all those miles walking have paid off. Even more curious is that there's not much in the way of blemishes and cellulite. My research tells me that those who have lost their weight on a calorie deficit end up with hanging skin. Not so with fasting. As the body chews into the protein, it regenerates skin cells. Or something like that, anyway. It's a process called Autophagy, which kicks in around the 36-hour mark of a prolonged fast. That's why when you see pictures of starved concentration camp survivors they never have saggy skin. Makes sense to me, although of course, they were *literally* starved against their own will.

But the principle still stands.

Once I'm done with my shower, I make the mistake of brushing my hand past the affected area on my hip. If you can imagine the action in slow-motion, then picture my thumbnail swiping down like a swinging ax and slicing right through the affected area.

Not that I knew it at the time.

It wasn't until I was flossing my taint (*"t'ain't the testicles nor the ass, but the bit between"*) that I clocked the streak of red, sticky fluid on the pristine, white towel fabric. I put the marks down to the fact I'm prone to the occasional nosebleed - especially in weather and temperature changes. Every summer and winter without fail. Perhaps I was having one, now?

No such luck. I accidentally sliced the affected area of my hip right open with my thumbnail a few seconds earlier stepping out of the shower. A few drops of blood had hit the floor. I look down to see the festering boil on my hip open and weeping with blood like some kind of burst volcano.

"Amelia!" I yelled down the hall. "Can you come here? Quick."

She made her way into the bathroom and nearly had a seizure.

"Oh my God!"

She whipped out a clean napkin from the sanitary drawer and caught most of the blood.

"It's my damn pants, I bloody knew it," I said in my British accent, hence my choice of words.

"You really need to see the doctor. This looks really bad," she said as she squatted before the offending area. She had a much better up-close-and-personal view than I could possibly achieve. "Seriously, first thing tomorrow. Tell them it's urgent."

"I will, I will," I said, hoping it wasn't something much worse.

A lot of what we coined "bad blood" had escaped. The swelling went down and that wonderful feeling of expunged toxins and nastiness from the swelling began. Amelia put a plaster on it. The adhesive used on the bandage appeared to have been made by a sadist, like it was made of wacky glue, and would likely de-root all the hairs on my side if I were to ever pull it off. Not wanting to tear the first two layers of skin off my side, I left the band aid alone, and cross my fingers that I'd be able to see a doctor in the morning.

Another reason to wake up early was because Beryl was due at 9:30 am for our regular, monthly clean. I am curious to see if she's noticed any change in me (and I'm not talking about my hip.)

So, an early night beckoned.

As soon as I finish typing the next paragraph I'll hit the sack and set my clock for 7 am.

Today is Kebab Monday (it's Monday, now) and I think that not-too-far goal is within easy reach.

Day 15, or:
"Kebab Monday"

*"Well, I don't want to get into a semantic argument over it,
I just want the protein, all right?"*
- Martin Q. Blank*, Grosse Pointe Blank (1996)*

<u>Monday, July 6th, 2019</u>

You may recall in an earlier chapter my mention of getting a doctor's appointment in the UK (whilst free of charge) being damn-near impossible on the day of asking. When you call to make an appointment you can expect to wait *at least* five days, if not more. If it's urgent (like my festering hip wound, which I suspect is infected) you need to get yourself to the hospital (still free in the UK, though for how much longer, who knows?) and get the offending ailment you have checked out.

There's a trick you can employ to make sure you get seen by your general practitioner *faster*, though.

The doctor's surgery opens at 8 am, and so I hit the sack a bit earlier last night so I could arise at 7 am. I had my morning salty coffee and allowed enough time to ensure I wouldn't have a pants accident. I dunno about you, but my general rule in life is to *never, ever* leave my apartment before I've moved my bowels. Fasting has changed all that, of course. As I drink my coffee and kept an eye on the clock, I realized I'd not eaten anything since Thursday night - 83 hours; which has to be some kind of record.

Anyway, the trick is to get to the surgery the instant they open and ask if they have a window free that day. You're physically present. It's way harder to turn you down. I set off at 7:45 am with the intention of arriving there on time.

And arrive on time I did.

The receptionist said to come back at 3:20 pm. It worked! While I was there I took the opportunity to weigh myself on their big, imposing weighing machine. I set it up, kicked off my shoes, and climbed aboard.

The result was... **14 stone, 7 lbs.**

I'd lost precisely *one whole stone* in fourteen days (14 lbs / 6.3 kg.)

I couldn't have been happier. Two weeks into what is surely a much longer process and I'd made a frightening amount of progress. It was all worth it.

Next up, my blood pressure. The results, thus:

SYS = 142 mmHg

DIA = 83 mmHG

PUL = 84 per min

My pulse was entirely on point. I don't know what DIA means, but my SYS - as advised by the chart on the wall - would ideally be 140, or a touch lower. I admit I was in a bit of a frenzy and didn't take the time to calm down before putting my forearm in the hole-thing. I mean I'd just discovered I lost 14 lbs and I was excited. But, what can you do?

I thanked the receptionist and said I'd see her later in the afternoon.

I returned home to do a few boring house chores, and couldn't stop thinking about my conversation with Shelley. If I felt the urge to tell her she could easily lose weight, then the urge to report my results to her was even stronger. I jumped back on my bathroom scales to discover the reading was **14 stone and 3 lbs**.

Bizarre, I remember thinking. According to the doctor's place, I lost 14 lbs. But my home scales are telling me I have lost 18 lbs.

Then I thought about my BMI results I conducted at the beginning of this whole process. I was slightly over / under the obese threshold according to two reputable sources. I swore there and then to continue corroborating any facts in future.

Today is Kebab Monday. I know you're dying to know how it went. All in good time, my friend. My plan was to have a light tuna and maybe a handful of cashew nuts to bring my stomach up to speed a few hours before my impending calorific Armageddon. I jumped on the computer and decided to find out just how many calories were in a typical doner kebab.

Doner Kebab with salad and sauce = 2000 calories, according to *livestrong.com*

Well, that's not *too* bad, actually. The lamb meat isn't fried, and, depending on the sauces you put on (garlic / chili) it can make it climb higher. It's all about the reduction of sugar and carbohydrates from now on - the focus being on protein and good fats.

Next up… a large fries with salt and vinegar = 510 calories. Of course French fries are just bad for you, period. But 2,500 (ish) calories didn't seem like much turmoil.

In all honesty, I didn't have long to wait. 8 pm was *massive* dinner coma-time, and that was less than twelve hours away. I mean, after a 90-hour fast what's another few, small hours? Besides, the tuna would roll round after I got back from Bean There, Done That, anyway.

I followed up my online research with a video from the renowned Dr. Berg who went on to tell me that one of the best ways to burn fast was something called Wheatgrass Powder Juice. A local health food store sells that stuff for £8 a go. It's right next to a music store that has a sale on. Okay, I thought. *Sure*. I've saved money on numerous takeouts. I deserve a bit of a treat. I'll go after I get back from my daily coffee routine.

And I'll walk in the blistering sun, too.

Walking on a 90+ hour fast must seem like the actions of a madman. Reader, welcome to *me*. I am mad. And I am a man, last I checked. Speaking of checking things, that wound (yup, upgraded from a mere scratch) on my left hip I sustained has really gotten worse. I put a plaster on it until the doctor can see what's up this afternoon. The chafing from my pants really isn't helping, and I'm about to do a four-mile round trip.

The walk to *Bean There, Done That* was awesome. With my earphones in and plugged into my antiquated mp3 player, I stormed through all the flats and hills thinking about my next book. I always do this. Music informs my ideas. It almost doesn't matter what genre of music I'm listening to. If it's hard and fast (like aggressive hip-hop) I think of action scenes. Slower and calmer music (Enya and Enigma spring to mind) perhaps something more tender might come to my mind. I confess, the thought about this very book being turned into a movie crossed my mind. I'm sure you've seen just how much of a movie fanatic I am by the chapter quotes alone. The idea of *The Hunger Diaries: The Movie* was fun, but then realized I'd ran out of visual cues to make it a success. How entertaining would a ninety-minute movie be about one fat slob losing weight actually be?

Funny you should ask that because - not ten minutes later - as I was crossing a particularly perilous stretch of road, a large truck nearly hit me at speed as it turned the corner. I stepped back onto the sidewalk in the nick of time. My razor-sharp alertness due to the fasting could very well have played a small part in that. On any ordinary potato-chip-kind-of-a-day might have made me more sluggish and inattentive? A post-lunch lull. Who knows?

Decidedly *unkilled*, I reached *Bean There, Done That* and had my coffee. The moment I sat down, I felt myself slowing down and entering into a sort of slow-motion hallucination - but in a good way. My glasses continued to slide down my face. The optician place is right next door, so I made a mental note to go there after I was done tripping out.

In addition to my salty black coffee, I have now taken to ask for a glass of tap water (i.e. from the faucet.) Now, I have two drinks - which makes booting the door open a bit more difficult.

I take myself by surprise when I realize that I am no longer looking at or judging others. *At all.* Short, tall, fat, thin etc people glide past my table going about their business and I don't even care anymore. I look down at my lap to see my belly doesn't bulge much anymore. Where my "titch bits" once acted like two, vast balloons under my shirt, they now seem to have at least deflated a little. I know this because my shirt doesn't get caught on them when I pull it over my head. These pendulous breasts of mine are still *there*, of course, but massively reduced (thanks, thigh master!).

I recognize a guy sitting a few feet away from me who I've not seen in a while. I know that face. He's chain-smoking and wearing a tee. It's *Stander*. Yikes, I've not seen him in a few weeks, and today he's *not standing*! What's wrong with him? Has he been given bad news by someone? Stander is sitting at the very same table Shelley was at yesterday during our heart-to-fatty-tissued-heart. Stander looks up and briefly acknowledges my presence, but I don't think he recognized me. He was probably being polite. After all, he usually has something of a top-down view of the patrons.

A lone guy in his late fifties is sitting at the next table, enough to see me *manspreading* and enjoying my new weight and body shape. He keeps looking at me for prolonged periods of time. Not wanting to cause a fuss, I avert my eyes to something big and bright yellow in nature. A stand outside the supermarket displays an offer. 24 tins of "Diet Soda" for just £7. As a former consumer of this devil juice, that's quite a bargain. No sugar, sure, but what about all that aspartame? It doesn't bear thinking about.

I thought I spent the first ten days resetting my taste buds. That was only partly true. What I was *really* resetting was my brain's interpretation of food. The good vs the yummy vs the bad vs the disgusting. Look at me. I'm drinking *black* coffee with a pinch of salt. If someone had told me just sixteen days ago that I would be drinking *that* and not have eaten for ninety-something hours, I'd have spat in their face and bedded their wife (if it was a straight, married male who'd said it. If it was a lesbian, I'd have done unspeakable things to their wife).

Damn, that peculiar guy sitting next to Stander just continues to stare at me. What the heck is this dude's problem? Who knows, but something needed doing. So, I do what I would normally do in this situation - *and stared right back at the guy's stupid, withered face.*

What you may not have gleaned about me from the preceding pages is that I am deftly skilled (with decades of practice) at two things:

1: Stare-outs. Seriously, you'll break way before I do, and…

2: Curse battles (impromptu or organized)

You read that second one correctly - *organized*. We did the latter *all the damn time* in high school when I was growing up. Two students taking it in turns to trade insults at each other for the amusement of a jeering crowd, all goading us into *hopefully* fighting physically.

You call me fat? I'll say something about your character. You call my mom a whore? I'll group your entire family together and suggest they did something *so* heinous, and in unflinching and worrying detail for a twelve-year-old who shouldn't know any better, that it'll make you want to barf. You call my dad names? I'll recall something personal you told me *months* ago - like your father being laid off - and suggest why that happened *and* mix doubts about his sexuality into the mix with such beautifully-constructed venom that you'll have no choice but to hit me to make it stop.

And resorting to violence is where you lose the argument, as far as I'm concerned.

That last one really did happen, one time. It was my friend, to make matters worse - who we'll call "Sam". I posited that his dad got laid off because he touched his manager inappropriately (that's the nice version, for the

PG-rated sake of this book). The crowd flew into an absolute frenzy, which prompted Sam to throw a punch at my face - and he missed. I returned the punch - *and didn't miss*. My knuckles connected with his jaw and sent him to the ground. Fortunately, he wasn't injured. I felt so bad and apologized immediately. He got up, shook the initial shock away, and we shook hands. All was well.

Secretly, I was happy that I won the conversation *and* the reversion to a physical fight. I've gone massively off-track, here. I'm not sure how it all fits into weight loss. Perhaps you recognize a bit of yourself in me, somewhere? I didn't exactly get bullied *because* I was a chubby kid. I got called names, of course, but that didn't happen often because, let's face it, if a skinny kid calls me "fat", then he's bound to have some messed-up physical or mental defect I can attack - like a wonky nose, a birthmark in the shape of the Mona Lisa on their chin, or whatever; you know, things about yourself that you can't change - unlike your weight. If I attack their character, it'll sting much harder. So, the instances of people calling me names were scant.

I thought about this as I sipped my coffee. That guy was *still* staring at me. I lost my patience (internally, of course) and stared him right back, but it didn't put him off. I mean, this went on for what felt like two whole minutes. In reality, it was probably twelve seconds.

Nevertheless, it was ridiculous. Stander (or *Sitter* as he's now named in my mind) was sitting next to him but hadn't clocked the stare-out. Enough was enough.

Still training my eyes on this guy, I let a small smile. He didn't return the favor. So, quite out of nowhere, I blew him what we in the antagonism industry call a "sarcastic and salacious kiss."

MWAH!

I followed it up with a cheeky, wry smile. Now *that* made him stop staring. He looked away, briefly, unaware of my new-found confidence (borderline arrogance, really) and weight-loss, and returned to my face and let out a pang of disgust. He collected his newspaper, stood up, and walked off, leaving a thoroughly-amused Andrew giggling to himself. Sitter knew something was up; that I'd done something to make the guy leave.

Thoroughly amused that I'd won a potential *gay-off* with a stranger, I walked into the opticians in search of my favorite pretty optician to tell her just how gay I *wasn't* by way of demonstration - and that my spectacles needed a good, hard seeing-to.

"Oh. You again," she mused.

"Yeah, guess what?"

"Glasses slipping again?"

"Uh huh."

She put them back in that machine *thing* again and gave them a bit of *whatever*. I couldn't resist this time - I asked what the contraption actually did. She told me that it's a heating device that softens the plastic so it can bend spectacles easier. I went on to ask if I were to put my hand in it, would it fry the skin off my fingers? She looked at me weird and said "no" because it's not *that* hot. Fascinating. I don't think things gets more exciting than that in this opticians, save for the girl stripping down to her bra and panties and *<Editor note: Andrew, no. Just no.>*

I put the glasses back on my clearly-shrunken head, and they threatened to slip almost instantly. The exquisite vision of perfection informed me that there wasn't much else she could do other than jump up and down on them and then try crushing them in her dainty, well-manicured fingers. At least I *think* that's the phrase she used.

Resigned to a lifetime of pushing my glasses up my face every eight seconds, I made my excuses, told her that whomever she was with was a very lucky man / woman / thing, and left the store with my index finger pressed against the rim of my glasses like a twat.

Walking home, I felt the urge to *slooooow* down. It wasn't nausea, though - more a feeling of tranquility. It was a serenity I'd seldom felt before. I walked slower than normal and just enjoyed the day. My brain was on hyper-alert. It was incredible, although I confess I did actually think I might not make it back home. Still, I soldiered on, and eventually got to the shopping mall near our apartment block.

My quest: buy some Blu Rays I can play on the massive 60" TV I'm going to buy for my office when we *finally* move to our new house, and get some Wheatgrass Powder stuff from the health store. I bought four Blu Rays I'll probably never unwrap, let alone watch, and I got the

green packet powder I was looking for, courtesy of Dr.
Berg.

When I got home I finally noticed the time. 2:45 pm.
Damn. I have about fifteen minutes to try this stuff I've
bought (not the Blu Rays, the other thing), and then I need
to get to the doctors to get my hip looked at.

The Wanker now has a new ingredient to be added.
Wheatgrass Powder. Here we go…

1 x glass of filtered water

1 x teaspoon of Turmeric

0.5 teaspoon of Wheatgrass powder

2 x teaspoons of apple cider vinegar.

Shake well in glass before serving.

Drink in one gulp…

… God *damn* it, that tasted like my worst nightmare. It
tasted precisely as you're imagining - like bleach mixed
with raw, used diapers. Another full glass of water and a
cigarette took care of the taste. If fasting seems an unlikely
proposition for you, then down a glass of that stuff. You'll
never want to eat again.

Thus, I give you the newly renamed cocktail of the
devil - *The Complete Wanker.*

Speaking of which… I just realized there and then that
I've missed lunch! I wanted my tuna to prepare my stomach
for tonight's death by kebab. But I might not have any

stomach lining left now that I've downed *The Complete Wanker*, and I have to leave for the doctor's now. Who knows how long I'll be? I'm certainly *not* going to eat tuna out of the tin with a fork as I walk because I quite like my reputation in this town. Not that I have a reputation, but you get my point.

Lunch will just have to be a thing of the past.

3:20 pm - Doctor's office.

"What's up, boo?" the cute, female doctor asked me.

"I grazed my hip a few days ago on that sticky-out bit on the door. And now it's all red-raw. It bled quite a lot in the shower last night so I put a plaster on it."

"Okay, let's have a look."

Doctor Woman (I can't be bothered thinking of a fictitious name) took my temperature, drew the curtains shut and ordered me to take off my pants. I did as ordered and removed the plaster.

She walked in and saw the wound and flinched.

"Oh dear. That's a bit bad," Doctor Woman said. "It looks infected. I think you're going to need antibiotics. We'll go with pills rather than cream."

"Are you sure?" I asked as I pulled my pants back up.

"Yeah, you'll be fine. Four times per day for seven days."

"Okay."

"And, Andrew, forgive me for saying this, but that's one of the biggest and thickest *pork swords* I have *ever* seen, and I mean that very, very sincerely."

Utterly unsurprised by her assessment, I sauntered over to the computer where she typed the prescription into the database, "Really?" I feigned, knowing full-well she was 100% correct.

"Oh, without doubt, Mr. Mackay. I'm surprised you were able to walk here. I've seen a lot of *curtain parters* in my time as a qualified practitioner, and yours is by far the largest."

"That's very interesting. I'm actually writing a book at the moment," I chanced. "Would you mind if I repeat what you just said in it?"

"Sure, as long as you don't misquote me in any way."

"I won't," I lied, before returning to what she really said. "Actually, in all seriousness, I have a bit of a weird question."

"Sure, go ahead," she said.

"I'm on a water fast at the moment. Is it okay to take the pills if I'm fasting?"

She stopped typing, thought about her response, and then stared at me like I'd just farted on her forehead. Pfft. The second person to give me the eye today. I didn't blow her a snarky kiss back, though, unlike that creep at *Bean There, Done That*. Twice in one day would be pushing it, and she's a not-unattractive woman. It was a different type of stare she was doing, anyway.

"Why on Earth are you fasting?"

"Oh, it's a detox thing."

"Hmm." She returned to the screen, presumably to add a note that the patient standing over her was verified insane and should be arrested the instant he walked out the door, "Fasting, eh? I have absolutely no idea."

I let out a semi-worried, "*Oh.*"

Seeming to not give much of a rat's ass about the fasting thing, she handed me the green slip of paper. "Here. Take this to the chemist next door. You can pick up your prescription, there."

"Thanks, Doctor."

"And good luck with that unfeasibly large appendage of yours, Mr. Mackay," she finished.

"I will, thanks."

I walked out of the building and headed for the pharmacy. The kind, elderly woman behind the counter took my payment and made me wait while her *unrealistically* beautiful Chinese colleague made up the prescription.

Pause.

We'll be coming back to this bit at the very, very end. It'll close the entire diary. Hopefully you'll see why I did this.

Fast forward to 7:30 pm.

Amelia got home and told me she'd read half of the book so far. She thought it was yucky, funny, and a few other things besides. She had concerns about some details of our life which I'm going to have to go and change. It turns out I've been *too* honest and revealing in places. Just stupid, little inconsequential things that might identify us. I hope you'll forgive my tampering with the non-essential details but I assure you that everything in this book is true.

"When are you going to the kebab van?" Amelia asked.

"Oh. I didn't have lunch today."

Amelia looked a bit concerned. "Are you sure you want to eat something like that after... how long has it been?"

"I dunno. About ninety-six hours, now."

"I don't think it's a good idea," she said.

"This is my treat, though. I've said this is what it's all building up to. I have to do it."

"It's up to you."

I must admit - at this point I'm as every bit concerned as Amelia is as I foolishly decide to go through with the kebab thing. I grab my car keys and some cash and make my way out of the apartment.

I can see the kebab van and its pretty "look at me" lights as I pull up on the quiet road. It's still daytime at 8 pm and rather warm, so I rolled the window down to let some air in.

The waft of burger meat and chicken hits me like a punch in the face. I'm *still* not hungry - not even close.

I end up parking a few feet away from the side of the van on the road. A line has formed. It hadn't gone unnoticed by me that most of the men and women waiting in line are obese - and that's being kind. One or two are not, of course. The smell from the grill floods the car. I find my senses are heightened, and hope my saliva starts flooding my mouth.

But it doesn't.

I'm not leaving my window open while I go there, so I wind it up and reach for my seatbelt, but my hand refuses to push the button and release me from my now-bigger seat.

To my astonishment, I let go, and just hang my head and close my eyes. At the risk of sounding over-dramatic (tough, it's all true), memories of the past two weeks come flooding back to me. Watching the Penn Jillette video. Learning about my body and the things that go inside. How fat-burning works, and doesn't work. How most dieters, like those on *The Biggest Loser*, failed quite spectacularly to keep the weight off due to a mangled metabolism. My wife feeling my body and finally relenting that I had shrunk and tightened. The time I farted watery diarrhea in my pants at the movies. How I nearly got hit by a truck. Stabbing myself with the door frame. The constant salivating at the beginning of the process. Figuring out how to prepare my meals. The liquid diarrhea I squirted because my stomach was empty. Endless spitting on my balcony. Being shocked at my BMI result. The same image of the obese individual you conjured up in your mind way back at the introduction.

I open my eyes facing my lap to see my belly had shrunk. My "titch bits" now much less of a issue than they were two weeks ago; I can now remove my t-shirt without catching it on them like a sleeve on a door handle. My skin - more vibrant and sparkling than ever before.

Finally, I thought back to this morning. One whole stone lost in two weeks. I'd done *so* well. No longer obese. I achieved my goal. I'm not man enough to admit I felt a bit of a lump in my throat - which was nice, because the last lump I felt was rubbing against my left hip and underwear. I can't deny that one or two tears rolled down my cheek. Not from upset, you understand, but from personal joy. How many times had I felt *that* in my pathetic, fat life? Answer: not often enough.

And then, my head lifts up to the kebab van for the final time…

***

I walk through my apartment door and make my way into front room where Amelia was sitting on the couch. She looked up at me and smiled, briefly, before squinting at my empty hands.

"Where's the food?" she asked.

I screwed my face nonchalantly and shrugged, "Ah. I changed my mind."

I sat at my computer desk and switched on my laptop.

"So what now?" Amelia asked.

"It's been ninety-six hours," I said with a great deal of chirp. "I think I can stretch it to Thursday."

"Thursday? A whole *week*?" she spat, stunned.

"Yeah, why not? I'll eat at 8 pm on Thursday. That will have been one whole week. And at the weekend we can go to *Thai Heaven*, our favorite restaurant to celebrate."

Knowing how much she loves food I knew she'd smile at the idea. Saturday it is. Just me and her and the Thai restaurant that acted as our first date. A meal that we love together, and always will.

"Oh, by the way," I added. "You'll never guess what that doctor woman said about my *pork sword*."

Amelia and I are about to go off and thoroughly smash Vow #7 to smithereens. You can't come with us, sadly. So, while we're doing that, you can keep reading and marvel at this bizarre and somewhat ironic denouement to the entire story…

***

Rewind… 3:30 pm.

There I am standing at the pharmacy counter like a useless fifth wheel on a quad bike waiting for my prescription. It didn't take too long. I wondered how the Penicillin might interfere with my prolonged fast. It destroys bacteria, which is definitely what I need for a small, localized infection. I didn't have long to think about it.

The pretty, Chinese dispenser girl glided from out of the prescription dungeon with a white bag in her hand, looking for its new owner.

"Andrew Mackay?" she announced, as if answering a quiz question about who the most handsome, slimline guy in the place was.

"Yes, that's me," I smiled.

She confirmed my address and plonked the bag on the counter, "I heard you have an inordinately large penis?"

"I beg your pardon?" I blurted.

She rolled her eyes and repeated herself, "I said… you must take four of these per day for the next seven days."

I exhaled, and thanked my lucky stars that the hallucinations hadn't started, "Oh. Thank God."

"You're not allergic to Penicillin, are you?" she asked with a gorgeous smile.

"Dunno. I guess we'll find out," I lied - because I know I'm not allergic but I wanted to make her smile.

"That's great," she said before remembering something important. "Oh, I forgot."

"What?"

"You *must* take these pills on an empty stomach."

There's no other way of putting it. I chuckled like an insane person at that line. It was as if the giant jigsaw of life all pieced together.

"Ha," I said. "That's ironic."

She shot me a mix of confusion and a polite grin, "Oh, yeah? Why's that?"

~ The End ~

Outtroduction

"I guess it comes down to a simple choice, really.
Get busy living, or get busy dying."
- Ellis Boy "Red" Redding, *The Shawshank*
Redemption (1994)

Well, we've come to the end of the book. What a journey!

I thought you might like to know that I am writing this *outtroduction* on Thursday July 11th at 8:40 pm. I weighed myself this morning. I'm now 14 stone and 1 pound (approx 198.8 lbs / 44.8 kg.) I have actually lost about 20 lbs in 17 days. Most of those days were spent fasting. You may remember I did a two-day fast, and then ate again, and have just now completed a seven-day fast. That is borderline *dangerous*. I know we're all impatient, but I really need to slow this process down. It's only mid-July, and I have under three months till my 41st birthday. There's that *gradual* word, once again.

As of now I'm over a third of the way in my pursuit of reaching my goal weight.

Most importantly, *I am no longer obese* - merely overweight.

I hadn't eaten since last Thursday. My water fast last one whole week - 168 hours without food. I went *deep* into ketosis and the Autophagy process.

In order to break my prolonged week-long fast I reintroduced my stomach to some food.

Wanna see what I had? Here, have a look…

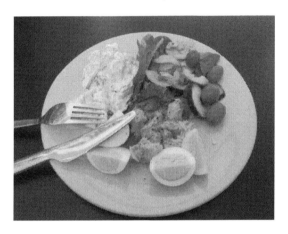

Two hardboiled eggs, salmon, spinach, four olives, some cucumber and onions, and a dollop of potato salad. Mostly protein and a hint of carbohydrates. Perfect.

I'm glad I ate a small quantity. If I overdid it, my stomach would have chucked it all back up. I'll sleep it off to prepare my body for tomorrow's lunch and dinner.

I cannot deny that I feel a bit devoid of physical energy. Days six and seven were *harsh*. Mentally, I was sharp as a tack. Physically? It felt like I was running on 12% battery power. Exercise was out. I had no choice but to just chill.

I should mention I am also on Penicillin - I just took my second pill of the day about half an hour ago.

Here's the thing I *need* you to understand. Do not ignore this next part. It wasn't until today that I realized why experts say that fasting is not for those who have experienced eating disorders (binge-eating, anorexia, bulimia etc) in the past. Amelia spoke about it early on, and it was news to me. The fasting process could *potentially* be addictive. You see results super-fast, and I just know there are people out there who will push, push, push until it causes them harm.

Don't let this be you.

Remember, the word "*gradual*" is your friend. I road-tested a two-day fast before I attempted this seven-day version. I'm being serious - DO NOT DO THIS if you think it isn't for you.

Now, if you are considering attempting what you've read in these pages, please remember the vow you swore by in the introduction. You fulfilled one half of the vow; reading up to the end of the book. But that last half? Consulting your doctor before you attempt any of this? No, you've not done that yet. Do not break your vow. Bad things happen when you break your vow. Consult your doctor first. If you are pregnant, a child, or have a history of organ issues (especially the heart and liver) or on medication of any kind, you *must* seek medical advice first.

As for the rest of you, I'll separate my key findings into an easy-to-follow bullet list in no particular order.

A Summary Things I've Learned, or:
"A Quick-Reference List"

- **Fasting is 80% mental, 20% physical.** You will have a few mental hurdles to jump. The physical is so insignificant when you compare it to the mental. For those of you who *love* food beyond all reason, it'll be a bit harder. With a pinch of determination, it can be done. It gets easier. Which leads me nicely into…

- The *Fool Yourself* method really works, too; far better than I'd given it credit for. From convincing myself that salt was sugar in my coffee, to eating low-fat beans and believing they were "normal" - it works.

- **Avoid weighing yourself every day.** Seriously, it's not worth it. If nothing else, it's not statistically significant. The last thing you need is to be put off on a Thursday because the scales reveal that you haven't lost weight since Wednesday. Remember, this is a long-haul affair. Weigh yourself once per week, *maximum*. It's a form of *Fool Yourself* in many respects. Just pretend you're losing a pound per day. The chances are greater (if you're doing it right) that it'll be true when you weigh yourself next week.

- **Telling nobody** I was fasting was a good decision. Amelia aside, I avoided the concerns my close relatives would have had, and the smirks and condescension I might have had from friends and strangers. The last thing you want is to be talked out of a decision. Fasting isn't well-known, and people confuse it for starvation. Naturally, they'd be concerned. I would've been, too, before I started this diary. Of course, with the forthcoming release of this book, *a lot more people* are going to know - especially if you leave a review and spread the word with your mouth and social media. I'm far enough into the process where I can demonstrate results (I'm thinner and not dead being a sound deal-breaker, probably) and potentially inspire others.

- **Eating nothing is immeasurably easier than eating intermittently.** It just is. Remember the last time you skipped lunch at the office, after you had no breakfast? How long did the hunger pain last? Yeah, exactly. It's entirely possible to go without food till dinnertime. So, a 16:8 (fast / feed) is very possible. You're probably doing it, already. My pangs of hunger lasted around 25 minutes, and then vanished. YMMV, of course. Trust me, though; it gets easier as the days go on. If you can't stand the hunger spikes just drink a full glass of filtered water. It eliminates the hunger in ten seconds, dead.

- When I finally break my fast tonight I just know that **I'm going to miss the sustained feeling of razor-sharp clarity**. It's like being on a drug. I've turned the anxiety and worry about fasting into a reason to keep it going until I reach my target weight. Never hungry, never sleepy. No post-lunch lulls. No need for afternoon naps. I can see why people of recommended weight do this. It's a sort of bio-hack where you can get stuff done much quicker.

- **Don't go to bed hungry.** Wait the 30 minutes till the period goes. Have a glass of water. Let the hunger subside, and then climb into bed.

- **Fasting saves time and money.** No takeouts, no trips to the grocery store, no food prep, no eating, no cleaning up afterward. You'll get through much less toilet paper. The list is endless. It's *astonishing* how many hidden benefits there are. If you're doing it right you might get used to not eating, which is dangerous. Be mindful of that.

- **Don't be afraid to research and adapt**. You saw this halfway through the journal. If I hadn't taken this seriously I might have ended up like those poor souls on *The Biggest Loser*. Who knows? Perhaps in the future another discovery will have been made. Stay up-to-date on developments as often as you can. This method of fat-burning isn't for everyone.

- **Do this for you, and you alone.** Don't do it because you want to get "beach ready" or "get into bed with that chick / guy" you like. It won't last. Think ahead for a moment - what happens when summer passes? What happens when you've laid / been rejected by said chick / guy? You'll give up, that's what. Don't become that guy / girl we all laugh at when they take out a gym membership in the first week of January, only to use it twice and then quit and head to Taco Bell to console themselves with a little cry over their chicken salsa burrito in the parking lot. If you do this for *you,* then the above examples will follow naturally. Remember the Roger Ebert quote in the introduction. It's 100% accurate. If you do it for yourself and your health, then the chances of you succeeding skyrockets exponentially.

- **Don't rush into the process.** Identify a time (maybe a week off work?) to road-test this thing and see if it's right for you. Do it when potential issues don't interfere with your work or life.

- **Weight and core training works better on a fast than cardiovascular training**. Sure, walk places and maybe go for a run, but don't go crazy with it. My legs (especially) are lean, now, for example. You burn fat on a fast (especially a prolonged one) when you're just sitting around watching daytime TV. Also, it's entirely possible to localize your fat-burning and "tell" your body where to focus on. Wanna get rid of those love handles? Do stretching exercises. Wanna reduce them "titch bits"? Use the thigh master and push-ups to get your body burning in those pecs. It's all about the core and building muscle. For heaven's sake, *take it easy and do it gradually.*

- **Think twice before you break wind.** After 36 hours, the chances are high that your stomach is expelling water in liquid form. You can hold it in until you find somewhere suitable to let it all go. Please, don't be a hero. In fact, scratch that; you should become that superhero Marvel have yet to invent - "*Bathroom Proximity Man / Woman!*"

- **SUGAR IS THE ENEMY.** Scorch this one into your retinas. It is to your body what water is to metal. Sugar turns to fat and stuffs it into your organs and fat stores. Insulin acts as a barrier and prevents your body from getting to your fat stores. Reduce your carbs to lower that barrier so your body can get burning the good stuff. High *saturated* fat and bad carbohydrate intake is the major contributory factor to you gaining weight. It's what gives you the "titch bits", the big belly, and the triple chin. Sure, the occasional milkshake or chocolate bar is fine; a modest amount will get your metabolism match-fit for the next burning session. Seriously, keep your intake of this poison to an absolute minimum.

- **It's not a diet. It's an experiment.** Diets don't work. Never have, never will. You know that. I know that. It's a journey, or an adventure, or a project, or… whatever the heck it is as long as it's *not a diet*. Let's just agree on this and move on our with our lives, shall we?

- Why not **write a journal documenting your progress?** It worked for me. It doesn't have to be *War & Peace*, of course. Just a small paragraph each night covering what you ate, how you adapted, how you felt, and the results. It's all be beneficial. Take it from me. *It works.* You're reading the evidence right now that it works.

- **Finally, you are not going to die.** Well, not with medical supervision, anyway. You must do your research. As someone who's writing this list at speed on 160+ hours of not eating, I can tell you that your body won't burn muscle. Or your brain. If our ancestors could go months without food, then so can you. Do it gradually, though (a 16:8, or *maybe* 24 hours), and see how you react. Don't be a hero and commence a 4,291-day fast when you close this book and chuck that Big Gulp and bag of Fritos in the trash. Someone's going to do it, though. I just know it. If anyone takes medical advice from a lunatic who (this book aside) tells lies for a living, then they deserve everything they get, as far as I'm concerned. Don't be a moron.

***

Well, I guess that's everything.

Before we get into the links I promised to furnish you with, I'll leave you with a list of excuses people have for *not* shedding those pounds. This is a personal list made by me and not researched in any way at all. Have a read and see if you recognize some of them?

Also, I have a very important question I'd like to ask you right at the very end. Frankly, I don't care at all about your answer.

But *you* care. Your answer is for *you* only. Make sure you answer honestly. Here we go with that list of excuses to not set about losing weight. Ready?

- I can't be bothered…

- My foot hurts due to a football injury, so I can't move much…

- I don't have the time. I've got so much work on at the moment, and don't have the mental bandwidth for it, even though I'd like to lose the pounds…

- I'll do it next week…

- Yeah, I'll definitely do next week - because my boss is on vacation and I'll have the water cooler to myself…

- Actually, *no,* wait. I'll do it on the first Monday of next month. Yeah, that's *perfect*. I can mentally prepare for it for the next two weeks. Yeah, this will definitely work…

- I own a Belgian Cake store in town and can claim what I eat on expenses. I'd be a fool to give that up…

- I'm already way too obese. This will never work. It's not even worth contemplating…

- I'm too old. Gaining weight in our later years is a given. It's not even worth concerning myself with…

■I'm on so many meds it's unreal. I don't want to bother my doctor about this fasting thing. He / she is going to think I've lost my mind…

■I'm still not sold on this fasting thing. I mean, I know Andrew lost all that weight, and the scientific evidence is all there, but I've never heard of it until now. Something isn't right, here…

■This is all well and good, but there must be a reason why I've never heard of fasting. I've not seen it in the stores and there aren't any commercials on TV for it. Why is that?

■Are you *seriously* telling me that I have to eat like a rabbit from now on and can only have artichokes and lettuce for the rest of my life? Screw that…

■Mmm. Hamburgers. Hamburgers chock-full with processed cheese and strips of beautiful bacon, topped with that special sauce. You know what? If I die, I die. Nobody's gonna miss me. I'm gonna go out with a massive coronary and a huge smile on my face…

With that, here's the final question I want to ask you.

Ready?

(Drum roll…)

What's your excuse?

Links & References

I don't want to overload you with too much stuff, so I've included all the videos and sites I consider important to round off the book in a succinct manner. These references - in almost all cases - were discovered during or just before the process and, without them, *The Hunger Diaries* wouldn't be the indispensable masterpiece it actually is.

The video selections have been very carefully cultivated by me for maximum, easy-to-digest information in as short a time as possible to get you started.

I've separated them into *essential* and *recommended.*

Now that you're done with the book *please* take an hour or so to dive immediately into the essential videos, now, while it's all fresh in your mind.

Some of them could inspire you, and some could even *potentially* change your life.

Essential Viewing:

1: "Why Intermittent Fasting Burns Fat Fast and For Good" (Bright Side, 28 June 2018) *(9min, 52sec)*

A must-watch. It tells you everything you need to know in under ten minutes.

youtu.be/Qngs_A2dnZ4

2: "Dr. Jason Fung - Therapeutic Fasting - Solving the Two-Compartment Problem" (Low Carb Down Under, 10 Mar 2016) *(36min,9secs)*

This is the exact video that changed everything six days into The Hunger Diaries. It put me on a different, "correct" track, and told me my original idea was wrong. I insist you watch this video. It's life-changing. I hold this video directly responsible for the success I had.

youtu.be/tIuj-oMN-Fk

3: "How Penn Jillette Lost Over 100 Lbs and Still Eats Whatever He Wants" (Big Think, 28 Sept 2016) *(9mins, 39secs)*

The video that started everything back on Saturday, June 22nd. I watched it, turned to my wife, and said "I'm doing this." Of course, we later learned that a calorie deficit and mono diet doesn't really work in the long-term. Nevertheless, this book wouldn't exist without this video and I'd probably still be obese to this day if I hadn't seen it.

youtu.be/NelIXCuuSZo

Further / Recommended Viewing:

4: "Joe Rogan - Doctor Explains Benefits of Fasting" (JRE Clips, 24 April 2018) *(8mins, 9secs)*

The video I mentioned on day seven's entry about fasting. Very enlightening, inspirational, and a major factor in convincing me I should at least attempt it.

youtu.be/bHdoAhZyP3I

5: "Intermittent Fasting: Transformational Technique - Cynthia Thurlow" (TEDx Talks, 15 May 2019) *(12mins, 44secs)*

Another video that compelled me to give fasting a try. This talk focuses on fasting for women in particular but is equally relevant for men.

youtu.be/A6Dkt7zyImk

6: "The Mathematics of Weight Loss - Ruben Meerman" (TEDx Talks, 11 Oct 2013) *(21mins, 25secs)*

Ever wondered what happens to fat when it burns? How it does vacate the body? This video explains how it happens, and if you reverse-engineer the fact, burning fat is much easier to comprehend and apply. Absolutely fascinating.

youtu.be/vuIlsN32WaE

7: "What the Winners of the Biggest Loser Look Like Now" (The List, 7 Mar 2019) *(11mins, 46secs)*

The sad inevitability of what happened to all but ONE of the contestants on the reality show. Now we know why this happened. Eat Less, Move More (i.e. burn more calories than you let in) worked great in the short-term. In the long-term? Months of getting it wrong utterly wrecked their metabolism...

youtu.be/KCrqUdnX3uk

8: "Why Long Term Fasting is AMAZING: 1-2 Day Fasts - Thomas DeLauer (Thomas DeLauer, 12 Oct 2017) *(9mins, 20secs)*

I've spent A LOT of time watching DeLauer's videos. It's how I discovered tips like adding Himalayan salt and Turmeric to my water fasts. If you're serious about IF - or prolonged fasts - I'd be surprised if you didn't YouTube-hop across his excellent videos.

youtu.be/Ojl9PｍｑAfhA

9: "Autophagy 101 - Everything You Need to Know - with Dr. William Dunn (Naomi Whittel, 13 May 2019) *(11mins, 48secs)*

Autophagy kicks in around 36 hours into your fast. As well as your body burning fat to survive, Autophagy regenerates your body by killing old cells and creating new ones. So, if lowering your glucose (which cancer cells feed on to survive), regenerating your stem cells, preventing illness naturally, lowering your blood sugar levels (and potentially reversing or preventing diabetes) and improving you overall vitality sounds like something you're interested in, then watch this. If it doesn't, just skip onto the next one.

youtu.be/ERKmJK_atdc

10: "How to Beat Type 2 Diabetes" (This Morning, 23 Sept 2016) *(4mins, 56secs)*

Dr. Michael Mosley - an exemplary authority on weight-loss - shows us which foods are good, and which are not, as well as a discussion about the 5:2 diet (5 days "feeding", 2 days "fasting")

youtu.be/7Ft6huxT644

11: "How to Burn Fat" (Dr. Eric Berg DC, 6 Jan 2017) *(23mins, 15secs)*

This is where I learned to add the final ingredient for "The Complete Wanker" (Wheatgrass Powder Juice) to my daily fat-burning cocktail.

youtu.be/ni5-3x6ofjc

Essential Reading:

1: "Obesity Overtakes Smoking as the Leading Cause of Four Major Cancers" (The Telegraph, Laura Donnelly, 3 July 2019)

Title says it all, really.

www.telegraph.co.uk/news/2019/07/02/obesity-overtakes-smoking-leading-cause-four-major-cancers/

2: "Why Are Americans Obese?" (PublicHealth, 3 July 2019)

I know it's a bit rich coming from a Brit but we're all taking North America's lead on pretty much everything, especially when it comes to the "size" of things.

www.publichealth.org/public-awareness/obesity/

3: "Childhood Obesity - Our Recommendations to the Nations (Royal College of Paediatrics and Child Health - Author & Date Unknown)

Written for the UK but, let's face it, it applies to any developed nation. A helpful laundry list of how we can tackle obesity for the next generation.

https://www.rcpch.ac.uk/key-topics/nutrition-obesity/our-recommendations-nations

Further Reading / Useful Information

4: McDonald's Nutrition Calculator (McDonald's UK)

Take a look at your favorite Maccy D items and see just how much fun your body will have handling it. All fast food restaurants have their own version.

https://www.mcdonalds.com/gb/en-gb/good-to-know/nutrition-calculator.html

5: BMI and BMR Calculator (Linear Software)

A combined tool I wish I had found earlier for the results in the book. Calculate your Body Mass Index to see just how much fat you're carrying, and the Basal Metabolic Rate to see how many calories your body needs daily in order to not die.

http://www.linear-software.com/bmr_bmi.html

6: "Super Size Me - Review by Roger Ebert" (May 7, 2004)

Ebert's review of the 2004 movie, which partly inspired this book. Contains the opening quote in the introduction.

https://www.rogerebert.com/reviews/super-size-me-2004

Fun Facts:

Calories in a Doner Kebab (or Giro)

https://www.livestrong.com/article/322440-how-many-calories-does-a-doner-kebab-have/

General calorie information (for large fries):

https://www.fatsecret.com/calories-nutrition/mcdonalds/french-fries-(large)

*All links present and working
at time of writing.*

A Word from the Author

Dear reader,

I sincerely hope that you enjoyed this book, at the very least.

Moreover, it is my earnest hope that it may have helped you consider your current lifestyle and possibly think about changing it for the better.

As you probably know, **The Hunger Diaries** was only meant for my own consumption. I never intended for anyone else to read it. It was about three-quarters of the way through the journey that I realized I had hit upon something that gave me real results… and could inspire others such as you, which is why I decided to release it to the public.

My editor (Aly Quinn) and proof readers have asked where my before and after photo is. The simple answer is… I didn't take a "before" photo because, honestly, I didn't think anyone was going to be reading these diaries. I can only apologize for this. I'd like to reassure you that absolutely *nothing* has been edited, altered, or fictionalized, as per my vows in the introduction. If you email me I'll happily send you a recent photo, though. Maybe you can compare it to my author picture?

"Amelia" wasn't especially overjoyed about her involvement in the book. She doesn't like nor deserve the limelight. That said, she saw the potential value in it when she read what I had written and encouraged me to release the diary in all its unedited and raw glory. So, it's her I need to thank again for compelling me to do all this. I can't believe how lucky I am, sometimes.

You're probably used to self-published authors putting huge adverts for their works at the end of the book. I'm not going to do that. **The Hunger Diaries** deserves better than that; it's my first non-fiction work, and without a shred of doubt my most personal effort. It's probably the one I am most proud of. Anyway, the book is peppered throughout with subtle and related plugs, so... all is well. (lol)

Of course, do check out my other works (it's all multi-genre and there's something for everyone) and follow me at Amazon to get an alert for all my latest releases.

I'm going to end with a heartfelt plea to you - and you probably know what it is, but I'm going to say it anyway because it's important to me:

Please leave a review for this book at Amazon.
Good, bad, or average.

Just two minutes of your time and a few, honest words is all it takes.

It will help a potential buyer to decide if the book is right for them or not.

Finally, if you'd like to contact me for any reason - whether you've been inspired to do doing similar, want to know how my continued journey is progressing, or just want to say "hi!" - then I'd love to hear from you. I always respond to my readers. They're the lifeblood of what I do.

I look forward to hearing from you, and wish you well for the future.

Andrew Mackay,
July 17th, 2019
"Chrome Valley", United Kingdom
Email: andrew@chromevalleybooks.com

Made in the USA
Columbia, SC
23 August 2019